69
WAYS
TO
LOVE
MYSELF

My Pussy's User Manual

YARETZI CARBAJAL LLC

© 2022 Yaretzi Carbajal LLC. All rights reserved.

No part of this book may be reproduced, stored in a retrieval system, or transmitted by any means without the written permission of the author.

AuthorHouse™
1663 Liberty Drive
Bloomington, IN 47403
www.authorhouse.com
Phone: 833-262-8899

Because of the dynamic nature of the Internet, any web addresses or links contained in this book may have changed since publication and may no longer be valid. The views expressed in this work are solely those of the author and do not necessarily reflect the views of the publisher, and the publisher hereby disclaims any responsibility for them.

Illustrated by Melisa Labra

This book is printed on acid-free paper.

ISBN: 978-1-6655-4811-3 (sc)
ISBN: 978-1-6655-4810-6 (e)

Library of Congress Control Number: 2021925833

Print information available on the last page.

Published by AuthorHouse 01/04/2021

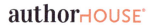

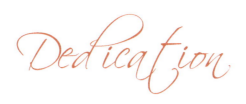

To my sisters:
The warriors and intellectuals I grew up with. I can only hope that you have learned from me as much as I have learned from you.

To my dear daughter:
You are a gift from God. My life has been filled with wonder as I watched you grow into the amazing young woman you are today. Never lower your standards—if someone loves you, they will rise to meet you at your goddess level of existence.

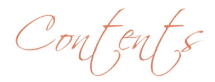

Introduction		ix
Section I	**Loving Yourself**	**1**
1.	The Case for Masturbation and Loving Myself	1
2.	Discovering Your Sensual Goddess	3
3.	Women - Warriors and Intellectuals	4
4.	Is Your Mind Preventing You from Loving Yourself?	8
Section II	**Flying solo**	**11**
	Waterworks	
1.	The Swimming Pool	11
2.	Jacuzzi	12
3.	Rigged Faucet	12
	The Amazing Pussy	
4.	Screaming Orgasm with Gardenias, Candlelight, and Mr. V	12
5.	If You Rub It, It Will Come	15
6.	Alone But Not Lonely	15
	The Self-Standing Dildo	
7.	Squats for Pleasure	16
8.	For Exhibitionists	16
9.	No Hands Required	18
10.	Trifecta of Pleasure	18
	Vibrators in Disguise	
11.	Microdermabrasion	20
12.	Mechanical Toothbrush	20
13.	Always Available	20
	The Food Section	
14.	Buttery Delicious	21
15.	Irish Cream	21
16.	The Always Hard Vegetables	21
17.	Chinese Eggplant, Hmmmm	22
18.	Chocolate – Serves Many Purposes	22

Other Ways to Love Yourself

19. Plump Pussy Cat and Its Forgotten Orifice 22
20. Go Fuck Yourself. . . . And Smile 24
21. Forceful Penetration (no, I do not mean unwelcome penetration) 26
22. Find a Way to Love Yourself 26
23. Start Treating Yourself with Love 26

Section III Flying with Your Lover 27

24. It Is Ok to Take the Lead 29
25. Warming Up with Mr. V 29
26. He Licks Because He Likes It 29
27. More Fingers, More PC Muscle Contractions 30
28. Add to the Activity 30
29. Squeeze Your PC 31
30. Suck, Lick, Bite Yourself 31
31. Accept the Feeling 31
32. I Ride, I Command 31
33. Lay and Stay, I Say 32
34. Bring in the Reinforcements – Mr. V 34
35. Bite Me . . . or Whatever You Prefer 36
36. Locked and Loaded Sex Rock 36
37. No. 34 Reversed with Butt Plug 38
38. Shower Poke and Swallow 38
39. Jane (from Tarzan) and the Towel Bar 38
40. Jane and the Confident Lover 40
41. Accountants are Underestimated Sexual Machines 40
42. Mobile Butterfly 41
43. Riding the Bullet 41
44. Ask and You Shall Receive 41
45. A Lover with Penis Control 42
46. Learn Your True Sexuality – Accept It and Embrace It 42

Section IV Flying with the crew of your choice 44

47. Allow for Experimentation and Evolvement 44
48. Be True to Yourself 44
49. Ebony Lust with a Fist 46
50. "He Who Controls Everything, Enjoys Nothing" 48
51. The Pussy Buffet 48
52. No Lover Left Behind 50
53. Find a Unicorn 50
54. Horseback Riding with a Twist 50
55. Allow for a Fetish 52
56. Pinned and Devoured 52
57. Silky Tongue Lashing 54

58. Banana Split Sunday	54
59. Double Fucking Renata	54
60. Dirty Dancing	56
61. Caught in the Act	56
62. Rumble in Booth #8	56
63. Chocolate Anus Lick for All	57
64. Exploring My Lover's Needs	57
65. A Step Further	57
66. To Fuck and Be Fucked (in unison)	57

Section V Set the Standards 60

67. Foster an Equal Mentality	60
68. Demand Respect	61
69. Education is the Best Equalizer	62

Conclusion 65

EndNotes 66

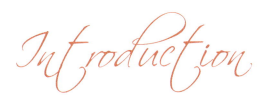

Introduction

For centuries, our sexual drives and motivations have been controlled and/or subdued through established societal norms, religions, and legal rulings. Women/females have been reduced to sexual objects, property, and domestic slaves under the presumption of being the "weaker sex." Consequently, women (and other sexual minorities) have suffered and learned to disregard their need for sexual expression.

Before I go any further, I'd like to explain that I am a liberal, heterosexual female, biologically equipped with female genitalia. My perspective is coming from a female born with a vulva, who was raised as a woman in a male-dominated, religious society. If I equate woman with female and pussy, and man with male and penis, it does not mean that I'm unaware of the other sex and gender variations. I am simply focusing on what I know as a heterosexual female with a pussy. This particular gender has suffered too long. It is time to free the pussy; it is time to learn its wonders and vulnerabilities. And, while I consider this a self-help book, I feel that this is merely the start of a conversation with ourselves. There are so many social and psychological constructs that we must break through to feel liberated. One little book is not going to get us there. I hope that this is the beginning and the reassurance that the raw, uninhibited, highly spiritual female (with a pussy) exists and is eager to thrive openly and unequivocally.

This book is the expression of my desire to help open people's minds. My purpose is to initiate an honest self-analysis about our true selves and our much-needed sexual/sensual development, which can, in turn, bring inner happiness and fulfillment. When we are genuinely happy with ourselves, we are less judgmental of others and practice empathy generously.

My love for human sexuality started at an early age, and my bachelor's degree in psychology grounded my desire to help in the understanding of our sexual needs. My practical knowledge comes from a sincere observation of sexual experiences and participation in the swingers community. I discovered that the sharing of loving experiences can help in our self-discovery.

I aim to stop the constricting sexual stereotype of the heterosexual woman that we tend to apply all too often. We are all unique, and the spectrums of sexuality, intelligence, and spirituality vary. My focus in this book is the amazing female who, if she breaks away from these social norms and obstacles, can achieve great happiness and self-fulfillment.

69 Ways to Love Myself is a tribute to all that can be achieved when you feel free to express your spiritual, sexual, and sensual self. Begin your journey to discover the superior female within and bring along your lover(s) who will enhance your enlightenment.

In this book, you will see the word "pussy" a lot; I like the word. I cannot think of a more endearing term for such a beautiful part of a woman. Well, I guess I could, but the names would be too long. Should I call it "the gate to heaven" …"the tunnel of bliss" …"the portal of pleasure"? For many of us, the term *pussy* means all of that and much more; the way to a woman's heart is through some awesome cunnilingus. So, get used to the word; know that its meaning is the most wonderful part of a woman. Again, please note that, to me, *woman* refers to a female with a pussy; I understand there are many other sex and gender variations but I do not feel qualified to write about them.

The main purpose of this book is to be used as a guide that will show every one of my female readers (and those who love them) 69 ways to love themselves. Keep in mind that there is no specific order of preference or magnitude. Since we are all unique, each reader will make their judgment of the sort. The first section establishes masturbation as a form of self-love, brings forth examples of amazing women throughout the ages, and discusses how our complex make up of hormones, psyche, and physical character creates our superior being. The next three sections are examples of self-love that are separated according to the people involved. *Oh! So, you thought that you would be doing this alone because the topic is masturbation? Not necessarily.* And finally, Section 5 focuses on setting the standards for how we want and deserve to be treated.

> **Section I – The case for masturbation and loving yourself**
> **Section II - Flying solo**
> **Section III – Flying with your lover**
> **Section IV – Flying with the crew of your choice**
> **Section V – Set the Standards**

Before I get into details, I would like you to equate masturbation to making love to yourself. Know that, like dancing, no matter the type of dance, there are the basic steps, the basic turns, the basic tilts that are the same. The variation, rhythm, speed, and ambiance make the difference. For someone to genuinely enjoy the pleasure of making love to themselves, they must feel amazingly comfortable with their bodies. Some need enlightening in this area but if you do not, if you are already there, you can skip the next chapter.

I AM

The sum of conflicting dynamics, a contradiction.

Frailty submerged in armor

Strength of character speckled with sensitivities.

I dream to be free to express all that lies beneath my composure,

yet I live aware of reality and fear I will never be understood.

A frail heart with tenacious mind,

I search for the one who will embrace my soul.

I search for the one who will love me whole.

Do not confuse my intention.

I call for you, not in desperation.

I call for you because we speak the same language of the heart.

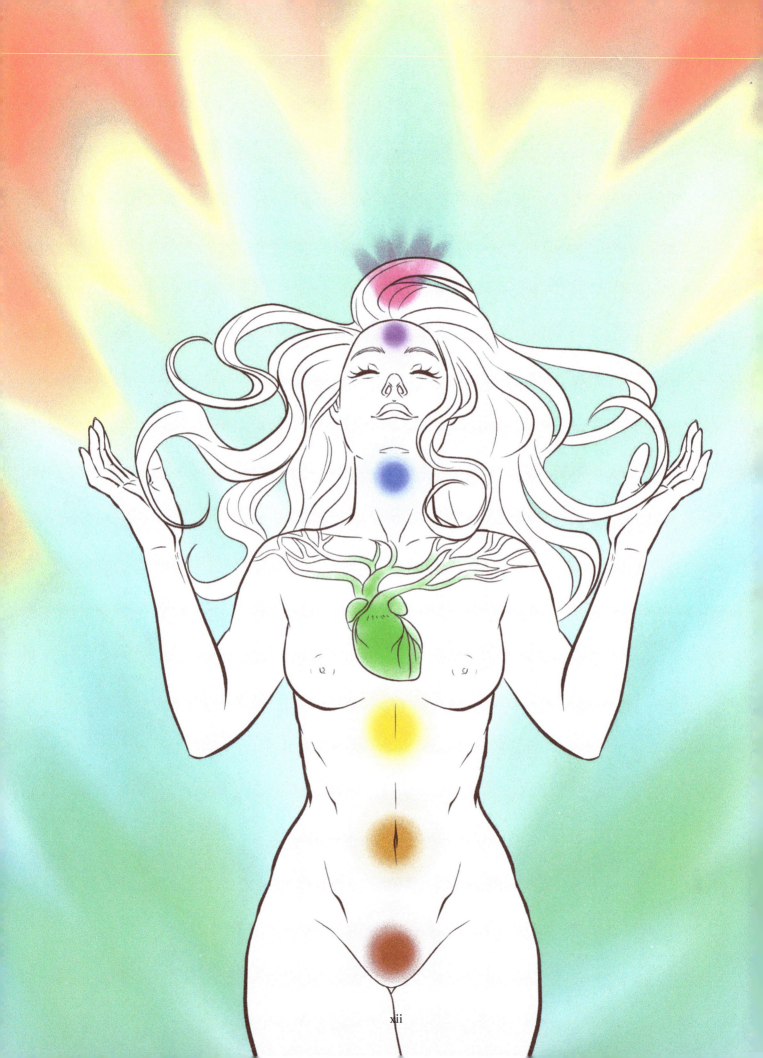

SECTION I
Loving Yourself

1. The Case for Masturbation and Loving Myself

As I finished screwing my coworker's sliding keyboard shelf to her desk, she exclaimed, "Wow, you are very handy with that," a comment for which I could not help but respond with the following: "Suzy, with a power screwdriver and a vibrator, you don't need a man." She almost rolled off her chair laughing. Due to her naïve, conservative-upbringing frame of mind, she thought I was kidding.

Ok, so I *was* kidding. Speaking from a heterosexual female point of view, we do need men. Nothing in this world can compare to the magical union of two beings, particularly if they join in spirit, heart, and soul as they love their bodies. My intention, however, is that we focus on ourselves and how we can experience love for our bodies, souls, and spirits—to clarify, the soul is our mind, will, and emotions; sometimes used interchangeably with the word "heart." Our body is the vehicle to earthly pleasures, and our spirit is our connection to the ethereal.

There will be times when we will be alone by choice or by circumstance. It is during those times when we need to care for ourselves; and, in the process, we have the opportunity become experts in our sexuality amongst many of our other facets. Masturbation is one of many ways to love yourself. If we know what pleases us, we can guide our lover(s) to the wonders of our bodies and reach a higher level of sexual satisfaction. We are also more open to new experiences that our lovers may introduce in our intimate moments.

Also, masturbation keeps our muscles toned; especially the most important muscle for sexual pleasure, the pubococcygeus (PC) muscle. Everyone has the PC muscle. It supports your pelvic organs and is responsible for holding urine and contracting during orgasm. It is placed from the pubic bone to the tail bone. Amazingly, in women, it is shaped like a slight curve that complements the usual curve of an erect penis.[1]

Remember that the same principle applies to all the muscles in your body. If you use them, they will be toned. If you rigorously work them, you will develop awesomely strong muscles. The PC muscle is especially important as it contracts when the pussy reaches orgasm. A pussy with a strong pubococcygeus muscle will have stronger contractions; thus, the lover's penis will be hugged, squeezed, creating a sensation that will drive it (the penis…and its owner) wild for a long time (depending on self-control). This is an important fact to keep in mind because hard bodies are not born, they are created. Your tight pussy is not something you are born with; you can body build it to WoW (Women of Wrestling) strength no matter your age.

The benefits of masturbating are mostly the same as when you are having sex with your partner: the increased blood flow, the calories spent, and the beautiful glow on your tension-free face thanks to the rush of dopamine and oxytocin released in your brain.

Dopamine, the pleasure hormone, affects through operant conditioning in our brain[2]—in layman's terms, an action that causes the release of dopamine in your brain sets up a "memory" connected so that the next time a similar situation occurs, a similar response will be produced. Operant conditioning is what we do when we reward our bodies with excitement and awesome orgasms when we masturbate.[3]

Oxytocin is another chemical that is found in our brains. It has been discovered that higher levels are found during orgasm and after, regardless of whether the orgasm was through self-stimulation or not. Oxytocin was first discovered to be released into the bloodstream as a hormone in response to stretching of the cervix and uterus during labor and with stimulation of the nipples from breastfeeding.[4] I strongly believe that the same reaction, the release of oxytocin, can result as we experience the stimulation of our cervix with a hard penis/phallus and the sucking and biting of the nipples at the height of excitement, and I found the support to my speculation. A study found that genital tract stimulation resulted in increased oxytocin immediately after orgasm.[5] Another study reported that increases of oxytocin during sexual arousal could be in response to nipple/areola, genital, and/or genital tract stimulation as confirmed in other mammals.[6] Murphy et al. (1987), studying men, found oxytocin levels were raised throughout sexual arousal with no acute increase at orgasm.[7] A more recent study of men found an increase in plasma oxytocin immediately after orgasm but did not reach statistical significance. The authors noted these changes "may simply reflect contractile properties on reproductive tissue."[8] My take on these results is that, concerning emotional bonding, women will benefit from the arousal of the male partner but not necessarily from the intercourse. Also, many men and women are often correct in assuming that after we enjoy intercourse, the female lover craves to cuddle. As research suggests, this is the time when the female's brain is filled with oxytocin. If you want her to bond with you, take advantage of this moment.

Oxytocin, characterized to be the "love hormone," favors the female body because estrogen has been found to increase the secretion of oxytocin and to increase the expression of the oxytocin receptor in the brain.[9] Since estrogen is a "female" hormone, this discovery made it clear why females can fall in love with the person they choose as a lover. The oxytocin released aids in the bonding; so even if we are not in love before we have sex, we become open to allowing that person to take a place in our emotional space. This is an amazing ability as it helps females in the selection of their mates. This is the gateway for the lover to travel from her body to her soul.

I have to admit that I have evolved in my thinking. In my early twenties, I believed I loved who I fucked; later in life, I believed that was a romantic's excuse to casually fuck without the consequence of being called a slut. Now in my fifties, I believe we are truly vulnerable; while we can select a mate and bond after some sexy fucking, we are in danger of bonding with the wrong partner. Thus, it is important for our young women to know this vulnerability and to be prepared.

Another amazing benefit of oxytocin is that it allows our brains more access to "creativity-related traits (e.g., novelty-seeking, extroversion, and openness to experience), and behaviors (e.g., exploration, divergent thinking, original ideation, and problem-solving)." Research has found a "consistent association between oxytocin and creativity, which emerges because . . . oxytocin enables the cognitive flexibility pathway more than persistent information processing."[10]

Back to Masturbation
Another benefit of masturbation is Classical Conditioning. This concept was established in the early 20th century by Ivan Pavlov. The idea revolves around the conditioning of an individual or animal to respond to a direct stimulus that is paired (presented) with an indirect stimulus. Once the conditioning has fully taken place, the individual or animal will respond to the indirect stimulus without the need for the direct stimulus. The important factor is to focus on a positive image of a person and yourself while you masturbate. For example, while masturbating you focus on your lover who has been away; by doing so, you are coupling good, sensuous feelings to your loved one. The more you do this, the more you will condition your response to his image. If you choose to focus on yourself, you will condition your body to feel good with yourself, and that alone is quite an accomplishment.

Back to the PC Muscle
Many have written and/or advised on how to exercise the PC muscle; however, exercising my PC muscle in such a methodological way is like doing aerobics without music. Get the picture? I prefer to have fun while exercising; therefore, masturbating is my preferred method for keeping the PC muscle in shape.

I do not want to indicate a norm of the frequency in which to masturbate—it all depends on your state of mind and personal preference. I can better explain with my own experience. For two years after my divorce, I did not involve myself with lovers; and for the first year, I had no sexual desire, not even to masturbate. Around the second year, my body started to yearn for the ecstasy, the excitement of an orgasm; however, I still did not want to be involved with anyone. Psychologically I was not ready, but my body was craving that awesome feeling. So, I went to my favorite adult toy store and stocked up on batteries and the basics . . . a vibrator and a dildo. At first, I used them several times a week; then my use went down to about once per week. As I became more satisfied, I did not need to use them but once per month. The frequency of masturbation depends on your state of mind and that is ok. As time progressed, I was more selective and expanded my collection; the right tool for the job is priceless.

2. Discovering Your Sensual Goddess

Through the years, I have read so much research about women being the "stronger sex" not only in the sexual realm but in other aspects of our daily lives. Women live longer,[11] have higher infant survival rates,[12] have a higher tolerance for physical and emotional pain, have demonstrated the ability to a higher intellect, etc.[13]

My focus, and amazement, is the sexual, emotional, psychic abilities all intertwined to produce a Sensual Female. But I do feel the need to explain the "stronger sex" reference. One of my favorite quotes by Timothy Leary (1920–1996) is the essence of this part of this book: "Women who seek to be equal with men lack ambition."[14]

When it comes to survival, male defenses are at a disadvantage from the beginning. In her article, Elizabeth Pennisi explained a Finnish study which points out that delicate male embryos are thought to be in danger of being naturally aborted during difficult times; it is suspected to be a "natural selection" mechanism to allow for female fetuses. The study of Finnish Church records of the 18th century demonstrated that the "typical ratio of 105 females-to-100 males" was unequivocally affected, and the largest difference was noted to be 100 females to 79 males.[15]

Scott Barry Kaufman Ph.D., in his attempt at "Setting the Record Straight," pointed out that, although women have lagged in IQ test scoring in the past, according to IQ expert James Flynn, women not only have caught up with men, women have slightly surpassed them.[16] His attention was to the operative words "women have slightly surpassed them." The emphasis was on the few differences which were explained as a "slight female advantage for characterological traits . . . a little female advantage because of temperamental differences. . . . They (females) are also more focused in the testing room just as they are more focused in the classroom." In essence, Dr. Kaufman agrees that women have surpassed men in IQ tests and explains that women have a "slight advantage." Moreover, the person holding the highest IQ score is a woman named Marilyn Vos Savant;[17] a reported score of 228 pushed her to stardom when *The Guinness Book of World Records* named her as the person with the highest IQ.

More and more women are choosing to reach higher levels of formal education. According to Liza Mundy in *The Richer Sex*, 57% of undergraduate degrees and most advanced degrees are awarded to women. Mundy makes a very plausible point of reversal of roles as women will take over the breadwinner title soon. My prediction is that women will also take the lead in the sexual realm. As women gain financial and political power, they will also have the confidence to court and date younger males who can keep up with their sexual needs.

3.   Women - Warriors and Intellectuals

When we remove, if it is possible, the chauvinistic, religious, and cultural norms, you end up with the raw, uninhibited, superior sexual, sensual, sophisticated female. Why do I consider her superior in the sexual world? Because women are capable of unlimited orgasms. Women can fall in love with the person they choose as a lover. Women have used their unparalleled cunning paired with spiritual and emotional intelligence to obtain unreachable objectives throughout the ages. This is true in all cultures, and yet, most have been buried in the past. It would have been very helpful to me to have learned about them as a young woman.

Empress Wu (February 17, 624 – December 16, 705)
I was overly impressed when I read about Empress Wu; she started as a concubine to the "warrior-ruler" Taizong and emerged as Empress within two decades. This was no easy task, but it demonstrates the beauty and skills she must have possessed to achieve this level of success. Even after Taizong's death, she skillfully positioned herself, first behind the scenes as an influencer and later as the ruler of the dynasty. And, while she was hated for killings under her command, during her reign, the accomplishments were innovating. "Her reign was peaceful and prosperous" while she advanced the place of women by "publishing biographies of famous women and requiring children to mourn both parents, rather than merely their father, as had been the practice hitherto."[18] There is so much more to this woman that would produce material for several books; this is just a very simple overview.

Queen Elizabeth I (September 7, 1533 – March 21, 1603)
Another famous woman ruler was Queen Elizabeth I. Surviving the obstacles before her crown was tumultuous and required amazing strength of character; perhaps this was the reason for her decision to never marry even

though she was known to have plenty of suitors.[19] Her accomplishments once she sat on the throne were many; these are just a few amazing accomplishments.[20]

Even though the young Elizabeth was rendered illegitimate when her father, Henry William VIII, had his marriage annulled, Elizabeth survived long enough to be next in line after Mary I fell ill and named Elizabeth as her successor.

When Elizabeth received the crown, she also received a bankrupt kingdom. She exercised "frugal policies" and established the Royal Exchange, which was essential for the "economic development of Great Britain."

Queen Elizabeth took on the discord between the Catholic and Protestant civilians by establishing England's independence from the Pope and cementing the middle ground with the "famous Elizabethan Religious Settlement."

Queen Elizabeth's leadership was a highly regarded determinant of the defeat of the Spanish Armada.

She encouraged more exploration to find more opportunities in trading and colonization (proof that women/females can also be cruel).

She gave tremendous support for art and literature, which opened the way for famous writers and playwrights such as William Shakespeare.

The pride of the kingdom grew as the arts flourished with peace and prosperity. This was due to the ability of their Queen "to keep England out of expensive wars and . . . able to crush conspiracies and rebellions against her, providing a period of stability."

Queen Elizabeth I "was a prominent writer and a great orator." This was perhaps one of the most needed characteristics of her make up. She was able to lead by inspiring her armies, her civilians, and the whole kingdom.

Cleopatra VII (69 BCE – 30 BCE)
Cleopatra was of Macedonian ancestry but cleverly learned Egyptian and molded herself as an image of Isis to win over the Egyptians. She devised a plan to sneak into Julius Caesar's quarters to seduce him and save Egypt from Roman control. After Julius Caesar's assassination, she seduced Mark Anthony and succeeded in being treated as a sovereign queen. She remained defiant till the end when she would not allow being paraded in triumph by the enemy; she chose suicide by poison.[21]

Enheduanna (2285 BCE – 2250 BCE)
Enheduanna was not only the first female author, she was also the first recorded author in history.[22] Her literary works—which referred to her faith, religious piety, and thoughts on the world and its wars—helped the people find commonality and a greater understanding for their peers. This was the goal sought after and welcomed by the King. Although she was named High Priestess by her father, Sargon of Akkad, she brought forth sophistication and higher value to the position for she was highly influential through her writings.[23]

Theodora (497 CE – 548 CE)
Her humble beginnings include earning her living as a wool spinner, actress, and prostitute. She became the Byzantine empress after Emperor Justinian I fell in love and married her. She became the emperor's primary

adviser and she improved religious and social rulings in her favor. Theodora elevated the rights of women and passed rulings to stop the enslavement and trafficking of young girls. She also modified the divorce laws to leverage more benefits to women. She was successful in ending the religious persecution of Miaphysites (another sector of Christianity) in 533.[24]

Mochizuki Chiyome (16th Century)
Another warrior of tremendous impact was Mochizuki Chiyome; a ninja that successfully recruited and trained other female ninja agents as part of the Takeda clan who served as spies, killers, and messengers in the 15th century.[25]

Juana Azurduy de Padilla (1780 – 1862)
Juana Azurduy learned to love indigenous peoples while working alongside them on her father's lands. Upon his death, her caretakers found her character too difficult, so she was sent to a convent with the intention for her to become a nun. She was expelled for the same difficult character at the age of 17. She later married and, with her husband, joined the indigenous revolutionary movement against the Spanish Viceroyalty of Peru. In the years of fighting, Juana devised a plan to extract the body of her husband who had been captured and beheaded by the Spaniards. She was also appointed as Commander of the Northern Army in charge of about six thousand men. Even Simon Bolivar is said to have recognized that Juana Azurduy de Padilla was the key to their victory; he thought the country of Bolivia should have been named "Azurduy" or "Padilla" instead.[26]

Harriet Tubman (Uncertain – 1913)
Born to the name of Araminta "Minty" Ross, Harriet survived truly horrible conditions, from severe beatings to fighting off pigs for scraps of food. After sustaining a severe head injury when she stood between a slave owner and the man trying to flee, Harriet often would fall into sleep/unconscious spells. This was attributed to her strong faith and religious beliefs. After she escaped to freedom, she returned to free slaves so many times that she became a living legend. And when the Fugitive Slave Act of 1850 was passed, she relocated to Canada but continued to return to help deliver more oppressed slaves to freedom. The conditions were unimaginably harsh. Harriet Tubman was one strong, determined, woman with an unbreakable spirit and unmatched cunning.[27]

Ernestine L. Rose (1810 – 1892)
A feminist and abolitionist, Ernestine was the first to petition the New York State Legislature to favor women's rights and to support the Married Women's Property Act, and did so at the young age of 28. Before that, Ernestine had already refused an arranged marriage, sued to obtain her mother's inheritance, supported herself since the age of 17 when she left home, and denounced religion because she "studied the texts of the great religions and concluded that all were irrational and oppressive to women." She lead the feminist side of the Owenite Movement (a socialist movement in England by Robert Owen) and, when she moved to New York in 1836, she was one of the first women to be an active speaker for women's rights. Her great orator ability brought the opportunity to travel to many states to speak on behalf of the women's rights movement.[28]

Ida B. Wells (1862 – 1931)
The young Ida had to drop out of school when her parents and a sibling succumbed to yellow fever. She quickly found work as a teacher (even though she had to lie about her age) in Memphis, Tennessee, to help her living siblings. Her outspoken spirit was stirred in 1884 when she was forced to move to a segregated

train car even though she had purchased a first-class ticket. She defiantly sued the railroad. From then on, Ida began to write and publish articles about race and politics while still working as a teacher until she was fired for citing the poor conditions of segregated schools. She later became the owner of two newspapers, and she continued to write about the terrorist tactics of lynching and the stereotypes propagated to rationalize them. Her investigative reporting exposed many of the wrongful accusations brought upon the lynched victims and even caused an angry mob to destroy her newspaper and threaten her life. Her numerous literary works brought attention to lynching at the international level along with the praise of famous leaders, including the abolitionist Frederick Douglass. In 1898, Ida took her anti-lynching crusade to Washington, D.C., calling for changes. She was a co-founder of the National Association for the Advancement of Colored People (NAACP) and founder of the National Association of Colored Women. Ida's courage, high intellect, and determination to attain a just government helped set an example to many future suffragists and civil rights leaders.[29]

Freddie and Truus Oversteegen and Jannetje Schaft (WWII – 1945)
Many more courageous women who stand out in a man-directed world are heroines of WWII. The ones who caught my attention were the Oversteegen sisters and their friend Jannetje Schaft, better known as Hannie. These astute teenagers used their sensual female qualities to lure Nazis to their execution. Hannie Schaft was killed just before the end of the war; Freddie and Truus lived well into their 90s. I humble to their courage, cunningness, and their love for the weak, for the latter was the main reason they turned to kill Nazis.[30]

I speak of women of the past who should have been honored and revered—little girls from my generation would have grown up aware of their capabilities. But that was not the case, and many women within our living generations have been fighting to elevate our status to an even playing field. One of the most "notorious" is **The Honorable Ruth Bader Ginsburg (March 15, 1933 – September 18, 2020).** She was demoted because she was pregnant; she was blatantly told that she would be paid less than her male coworkers in similar positions because she was married; she could not find a job even though she had graduated from Harvard and tied first in her class. And back then, it was a legal practice. However, this petite but steeled character was able to slowly chip away at the discriminatory laws between the genders. She ingeniously found male clients that were on the losing side of the law and demonstrated that treating genders differently hurts everyone. Thanks to her perseverance, women and men can enjoy equal protection under the law. This major achievement opened the door to a torrent of other cases including institutions such as the IRS for rulings of equal caregiver deductions, the military for equal housing allowances, and later the Social Security Administration for equal survivor benefits. RBG strategically challenged involuntary sterilization the same year Row vs. Wade was fought in court. She later fought against different legal drinking ages for men and women. She fought for the right to jury duty for women. As a judge, she continued cementing the 14th Amendment to "strike down the Virginia Military Institue's male-only admission." Her contributions are too many to list here.

We currently have so many amazing women who are fabulously smart, relentless, and resourceful; it is our duty to keep their accomplishments alive and expose our sons and daughters to their achievements and contributions to society.

Malala Yousafzai (born July 12, 1997)
A more recent example of a courageous woman is the very young Malala Yousafzai. As Naomi Blumberg describes in her article "Malala Yousafzai Pakistani Activist," Malala was a Pakistani teen who protested the prohibition of education of girls. The world noticed her struggles when she was shot in the head in

an assassination attempt by the Tehrik-e-Taliban Pakistan or TTP in October 2012. She proved to be unstoppable. In July 2015, she opened a girl's school in Lebanon for Syrian Civil War refugees. In 2014, She was awarded the Nobel Peace Prize for her fight to the right for education to all children, including young women.[31] And on June 19, 2020, Malala Yousafzai graduated from Oxford University with degrees in philosophy, politics, and economics.[32]

Tarana Burke (Born September 12, 1973)
She started the #MeToo movement in 2006 to help women survivors of sexual abuse heal.[33] Since then, this movement has taken off and has been instrumental in bringing light to the dynamics of the social construct that allows for sexual abusers to thrive.

Greta Tintin Eleonora Thunberg (Born January 3, 2003)
Greta is a young activist fighting to reduce our carbon footprint and thus reduce climate change, which is dramatically increasing. In August 2018, she started her public activism outside of the Swedish parliament calling for actions to reduce climate change. She has proven to be a strong voice for the young people who have realized that they need to be a part of the change if they want a hospitable world to live in; this movement has been called "the Greta Effect."[34] Strong in her conviction to reduce carbon emissions, she chose to sail across the Atlantic to attend the UN Climate Action Summit in 2019.[35]

Alexandria Ocasio-Cortez (born October 13, 1989)
The Congresswoman cordially dubbed as AOC won her seat in the House of Representatives in 2018, and since then she has taken Congress by storm with her progressive and ambitious agendas. She served as a great example of a woman facing the struggles of a culture dominated by the heterosexual male when she took on a colleague for calling her a "fucking bitch" on July 21, 2020. His intellect had no recourse when discussions and debates in Congress were difficult to beat, and he could not intellectually match her argument. In her speech on the House of Representatives floor two days later, AOC put the national spotlight on the culture that insults, dehumanizes, and seeks to control women, especially women who they consider "dangerous"— "they" are those who align to this culture referenced above. And, while this may not seem a great achievement in comparison to other women mentioned, AOC is a force to be reckoned with and will continue to strive for a better world. "They (my parents) did not raise me to accept abuse from men" is a phrase that we need to engrain in our daughters' brains from early childhood.[36]

There is an astonishing number of women in history who have accomplished great feats, strong women who did not accept their society's standards, yet we are barely learning about them. Unfortunately, early in our Human history, women were oppressed into second class citizens and most of them degraded to mere objects for sexual pleasure for men. But strong women and their strong movements are again leading a trend to improve the treatment of women in our culture. With all the research now available, women have woken up to the indisputable realization that, the raw, uninhibited, sexual, spiritual female is a superior, highly evolved being. She is in touch with all senses and beyond which allows her to fully open to receive the male spirit on an equal field and blend as one. Few men have reached that level of spirituality; thus, women are left out at this higher level without a mate.

4. Is Your Mind Preventing You from Loving Yourself?

You are a sensual female spirit, and if you do not feel it yet, the next step is to get to the bottom of the reasons your mind is giving you. Find out why you are giving yourself such an erroneous attitude about you, the real you. Yes, it is easier said than done. I should know. Around the age of thirteen, I encountered what psychology professionals call an inferiority complex. Coming to this country from Mexico, knowing only the most popular words in English (yes and no), I quickly learned to read and was lucky to invest my love for reading in the self-help genre. For about a year, I was too shy to face the crowd in the school cafeteria, so I would sneak in food to eat while consuming the self-help section of the library. I strongly believe that by knowing yourself, you learn to love and heal yourself, which will drive you to respect yourself. My love for myself was again tested in my late twenties when I started to lose my hearing. I can frankly tell you that I know how one feels inferior during such experiences. I have been there. Not everyone has the opportunity for psychotherapy but, if you do have the opportunity to counsel with a professional, please do. But keep in mind that any change is a process; it will not happen overnight, so the first thing to do is to exercise patience with yourself.

Not so long ago, a wise gentleman with an aura similar to that of a Yogi monk wrote to me: "look for what you need inside you because you have it." This phrase has now become part of my internal drive. I remind myself anytime I start to feel the need for encouragement, and I realize now that this book reflects that ideal. There is so much within us that fulfills most of our needs. Do not confuse my message. I am not inferring that we do not need a loving partner in our lives. Some people need several loving partners (polyamorous), some only need one but have the kinky need to share sexual experiences (swingers), and some only need one for themselves (classic monogamous ideal). My message, which was my friend's message, refers to all that we have inside, which is our true guidance and true love. If we become aware of our true beauty and talent, then we can coexist with our loving partner(s) without making them responsible for our happiness, for happiness is within us.

When I say to treat yourself right, I also mean to stop sacrificing your health over getting a few more tasks accomplished. A few decades ago, I experienced constant constipation. I tried laxatives, but they only perpetuated the situation. It took me a while to realize that I had brought that condition on to myself, my body. My internal drive is to be productive. I learned early on that my culture valued me depending on how much work I produced; thus, in constant motion, I filled my life with little projects in addition to having to work for a living. I have always taken pride in being fast, efficient, and industrious—nothing wrong with that, right? Well, no, but I pushed myself so much that I would not take the time to go to the bathroom and relax when I had to allow my bowels to do their duty. Once your body keeps your poop too long it excretes more water from the feces making them rock hard and difficult to move out. Then the laxatives move everything out, including nutrients from the food you just consumed, but most damaging is that your muscles that help in the movement of your bowels lose their strength over time. I have learned to give my body the time it needs because I love my body, and that is an extension of the love for myself. The same applies to my habit of eating while multi-tasking. I realize that now, but I still must work through it.

Learning to love yourself is a process. The process begins when we learn to love from the people around us in our early years. It expands when we learn to educate ourselves. There comes a time when we know we need to expand our conceptual horizons. Some are lucky to have learned healthy ways to love; however, the cultural norms have taught women to put their needs aside for their men and children. Therefore, we must educate ourselves about love and self-love with up-to-date information.

In her article "Learning to Love and Be Loved," Dr. Roni Beth Tower, Ph.D. listed the necessary ingredients to learn to love ourselves as curiosity, attention (to ourselves), compassion, and acts of kindness. Armed with those ingredients, we can begin our journey to actualize our concept of self-love.[37]

Coincidentally, all of those ingredients are part of this book. We have to have great curiosity to want to know ourselves. We must pay attention to our bodies and emotions as they react, positive or negative, to a stimulus. We must be empathetic for our concerns and address them, and acts of kindness to ourselves such as removing negative influences and unhealthy habits are essential. All of these ingredients must be present to move forward because it is true that we cannot love others (in a healthy way) until we love ourselves.

Once you reach the point of loving yourself while acknowledging that you are not perfect, a new world opens to you. You choose your mate, you choose your friends, career, workplace, etc. You also have the strength to be alone when you choose. You choose to relate to loving, supporting people around you, and you distance yourself from the negative influences even when they tell you they love you, even when they call themselves "friends."

Once you love yourself, you can look in the mirror and see the sensual woman I am referring to. Whether you have full, succulent breasts, or small with perky nipples enticing a bite; or strong thighs with full pussy lips that cover a thriving clitoris; just as sexy, a thin body frame with a small waist that men would love to hold while thrusting from behind. You are a goddess with more power than you realize. Nevertheless, it is a positive force that you can harness to make your intimate world a much sexier place. And keep in mind that, when I refer to our "superior being," I mean that we are superior in comparison to what we were raised to believe in this male/Christian-dominated society. No human being is superior to another one. I am simply bringing to light that too many women were raised to behave as second-class citizens.

SECTION II
Flying solo

The first 23 ways to love myself are examples of a journey that many of us embark on while weighted down with insecurities. As mentioned earlier, I equate masturbation to a form of self-love. Nurturing this self-love is essential for our psychological health. It is important to note that masturbation is not the only way to love ourselves, but it is my focus here.

At an early age, I discovered that a controlled flow of water with a certain amount of pressure onto a certain spot on your body could give you the purest pleasure. Something happened to the showerhead, but I still had to take a bath or shower. I opted to shower seeing it as the fastest way to comply with my mother's orders. In the middle of my shower, I laid down to let the water cool me down. I was extremely hot and tired from playing—lucky me. As I laid down, the water streamed right in between my legs. I was amazed by the pleasure; so pure, so simple, so natural.

The idea of writing this manuscript came to me while I was in the pool. Water has always been a sensual element in my life. I can feel the bodies exchanging mystical vibes with less resistance. It acts as a transmitter, and for that reason, I prefer to be in the pool only with people I know and love. A long time ago I discovered the fabulous pool water jets that keep the water circulating. Since then, I go back to them to revisit that feeling. If the pool is a public or semi-public, the risk of being seen may affect your pleasure. Some people get more excited about the danger of being seen, while others would be terrified.

Waterworks

1. The Swimming Pool

Pull yourself very close to the water jet and lift your leg (or legs if you can) while holding on the edge. Let the pressured water flow straight to your bikini area. It may take a while, but once you feel that warm feeling and sensation over your pussy, pull the bathing suit to the side with one hand while still holding on to the edge with the other. Feel the full force of pressure over all your pussy lips, clitoris, and the entrance to your vagina. In no time, your pussy will be so engorged and sensitive that you will come.

2. Jacuzzi

For more private moments, a Jacuzzi is the next best thing. Same principle: position yourself to where the water jets on to your vagina but do not open your lips yet. Let the insinuating vibration massage it until you can feel you're engorged. Once you need to, pull your lips apart with your index and middle finger. Keep indulging yourself then tilt a bit so that the water jets onto the entrance to your vagina. If successful, you will feel like you are being penetrated.

3. Rigged Faucet

I removed the faucet from my bathtub; I did not like it at all. I did not replace it. I am incredibly happy with my water pipe which sends the water on a pressured jet straight out but then starts falling on a curve like a stream. At the end of that stream, yes, you guessed it; my eager pussy lays there on occasions. Same principle: the water sends vibrations throughout, each time covering more of me. After a while, my pussy begins to feel so engorged; it grows as the sensation and vibrations grow. At that moment, I open my lips and let the pressure travel to the vaginal orifice. The pressure maximizes my pleasure, and I begin contracting, reaching orgasm.

But enough about waterworks; let us move on to my favorite topic of power tools. Again, a long time ago I learned that power tools can be a girl's best friend because we can get the job done faster with professional precision and magnitude. I have remodeled one kitchen, I'm in the process of remodeling another one and do much of the repair work in my residential rentals. I highly value the right tool for the right job. I also know that sometimes you must be resourceful and use tools in a way they may have not been intended but that will satisfy your specific needs. More importantly, the combination of tools to do the job is often a better way to do things. Still, with all the wonderful tools at hand, knowing your body is essential to please yourself.

The Amazing Pussy

4. Screaming Orgasm with Gardenias, Candlelight, and Mr. V

Picture in your mind lying on cool, soft cotton sheets with the scent of Gardenias, dim candlelight, and soft seducing music of your choice. Your favorite vibrator (Mr. V) begins to hum while you watch those sexy bodies on a pornographic video. You use the slow setting to give yourself time to wake your senses. As your pussy swells and you smell the precious musky scent of your body cream, you increase the speed because you are ready for more. Louder is the humming of your stoic companion, and so delightful are the vibrations it sends throughout your now engorged pussy. Second by second, the vibrations encompass more of you and the soles of your feet come together while your thighs are fully spread like butterfly wings. Amazingly, you become so flexible that your pussy is completely open. Your lips are so wet and your clitoris has never been as big. At this moment, take one finger (not from the hand holding the vibrator, keep it going) and VERY SLOWLY insert it in your vagina. Insert only the tip of your finger (the nail part down) with the pad facing up (index finger works best in my experience). Now keep going in and out taking care that no more than one inch of your finger goes inside you. Keep doing this slowly until you feel the urge to speed up. Your finger will soon feel hugged by your silky wet pussy. You will feel your temperature rise and the amazing sensation will be so intense that you will want to stop . . . but DO NOT STOP. Keep going until you cannot help but moan, even scream. Congratulations! You have just given yourself a screaming orgasm.

A particularly important lesson to be learned is that you do not have to go too deep into a woman's vagina to make her feel pleasure. You also do not have to be very thick to make her squirm in orgasmic delight. You only need the right spot, rubbing at the right speed, at the right moment. This spot is located within your vagina right behind your clitoris . . . some call it the G-spot; I call it the backside of my clitoris. Also take note that porn videos may not be necessary, and for some, it may hinder the sensual feeling. I recommend trying with and without videos; that is the only way to know if it works for you.

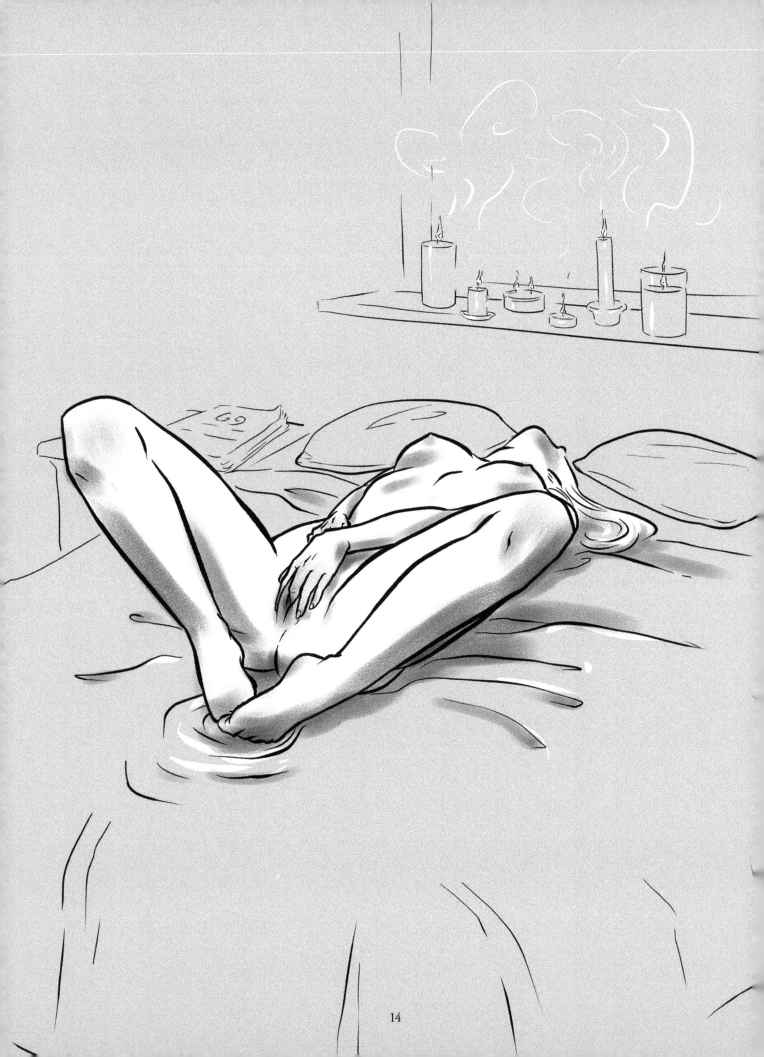

5. If You Rub It, It Will Come

If #4 was too much for your taste, then try a more natural, sensual way. Take time after you've showered and feel so clean that you can smell the freshness in the air. Rub body lotion or oil all over and spend more time wherever it pleases you. Your breasts, for example, are also sensitive to sensual stimulation. Grab them with both hands and slightly massage. Feel your nipples with the tips of your fingers. Take time to get to know that part of you. Feel the soft nipples grow hard denoting your excitement. If you have big breasts that you can pull towards your mouth and take a small bite, go ahead…or just lick, suck, whatever you prefer. Keep feeling your breast(s) with one hand and bring the other hand to the top of your pussy just over the crevice (just above the clit). With fingers facing down, softly move them together in a circular motion. This will slowly send vibrations to your clitoris. It will take longer than other forms of masturbation because it is done indirectly; however, you will start feeling that excitement in your pussy soon enough, along with the flow of your natural lubricant. Keep rubbing. You may change the direction of the movement if you wish. The idea here is "if you rub it, it will come."

For some of us, this form of masturbation would test our patience. However, after being exposed to vibrators, we may overlook the especially important concept of delayed gratification. Slow loving can be so hypnotic, and the strength of your orgasms will still be as potent. The pleasure of feeling penetrated will never go out of style . . . therefore, a dildo is just as necessary as a vibrator. Some tools have incorporated both into one, but my personal preference is to use each to complement the other.

6. Alone But Not Lonely

A couch by the window overlooking a garden; a glass of wine and lace to make you feel sexy inside and out. It has been a long time since your last encounter with a lover. Nevertheless, you are not about to squander your delicate sensuality over a casual, callous fling. When you can love yourself, you build up the strength to wait for the right person. Feeling so sexy with your legs now wide-open sitting on that couch, you begin to touch you, feel you, and even kiss your breasts. The feeling only intensifies as you bring the vibrator to your eager pussy so ready to feel alive again. The vibrations, even in the slow setting, cause your pussy to drip—it is soaked with your natural bodily secretions. Continue probing yourself as you wish. Then, as you reach a certain point of excitement and your pussy is contracting but not because of orgasm—contracting as if calling, screaming to get penetrated. You reach for your dildo and bring its head right to the opening of your vagina. While you keep your vibrator on your clit, you tease yourself and slowly penetrate yourself. Slow is the key until you reach ecstasy. Then, only then, you speed up your hand moving the dildo in and out, in and out, till your hungry pussy is satisfied.

Active women may prefer a more strenuous form of enjoyment that can be achieved by being on top. A dildo was made specifically for such purpose. The shaft end is shaped for suction so that as it is pushed against the floor, the kitchen counter, bathtub, etc., it will stay in place, which is very useful for the next forms of masturbation.

The Self-Standing Dildo

7. Squats for Pleasure

A cool shower was on my mind, but the South Texas sun overheating my pussy when I tanned got me to craving some physical thick thigh loving. You can achieve sexy strong thighs when you practice this often. Place the dildo on top of the bathtub wall so that you can hover over it by placing one foot in the tub and the other on the outside of the tub. Start with the mild setting on your vibrator, placing it gently over your pussy. As you begin to feel the wet excitement, speed up to the next level and right before your pussy starts contracting, slowly squat till you feel the head of the dildo penetrating you. Go up and down, but do not go too deep (unless you prefer it). It is my experience that at first, shallow penetration can be more exciting.

8. For Exhibitionists

If you're an exhibitionist, set the dildo on top of a small table or chair in front of a mirror. We tend to close our eyes when feeling intense excitement, but try looking at your pussy. See how it devours that dildo. Seeing your sexual hunger may add to the excitement. Only by trying it can we can find out if we like watching ourselves and dare to be our own audience. The great benefit of being on top and squatting is the wonderful exercise you give to your thighs and buttocks. Also, as gravity pulls your insides down it makes your pussy feel slightly tighter.

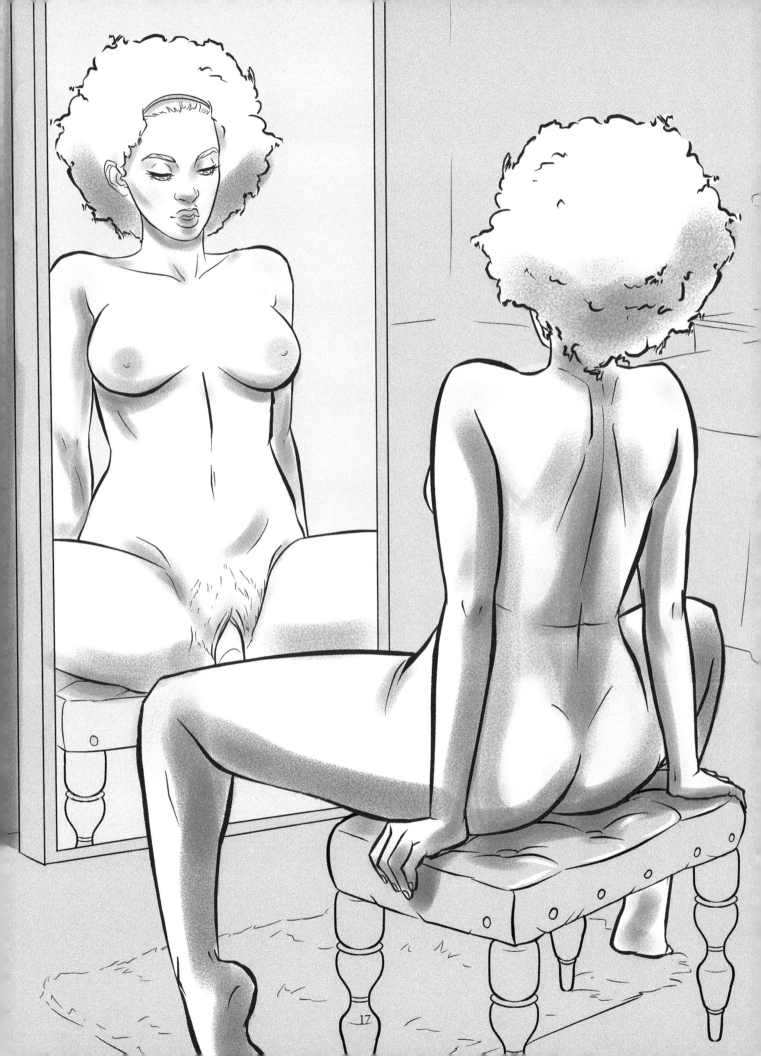

9. No Hands Required

On other occasions, while doing #7 or #8, add to this a butterfly vibrator. This is the best choice for this situation because it straps onto your pussy, continuously sending those amazing waves of pleasure to your clitoris while you ride that dildo at your desired pace. (Note that this is the original butterfly, which is only a vibrator, not the latest version with G-spot penetration). Ride high, ride low, ride, ride, ride till you come.

10. Trifecta of Pleasure

Take this #9 experience one step further into ecstasy. Rub some lubricant at the tip of the erect dildo, step over it while you feel so high from the vibrating butterfly humming over your pussy. At that point of extreme pleasure where your pussy is contracting eager to swallow that cock, insert the tip of your index finger. . . yes, it feels so hot that you are ready to come, but wait . . . keeping your finger in your pussy, slowly squat down and guide (if necessary) the tip of your dildo into your anus. Start slow and let your desire guide you. This is what I call the trifecta of pleasure. Our bodies can feel intense pleasure from three places: the clitoris, vagina, and anus. You are a true goddess of sensuality; your body was made for the physical pleasures maximized with your feminine intuition and sensitivity.

For some, anal penetration is not even conceived, while for others it is just one more way of enhancing the sexual experience. I discovered late in my 40s that anal penetration can be a pleasurable experience. This is a bit late in life compared to some women, but my first experience, in my early 20s, was painful and after that I was afraid. Thanks to a very gentle lover, I agreed to try again, and it was incredible. I learned that, for me, it is not something to do every single time I have sex. I discovered that I must be extremely excited to crave and enjoy anal penetration. The audacious willing to experiment will learn their true sensual/sexual character.

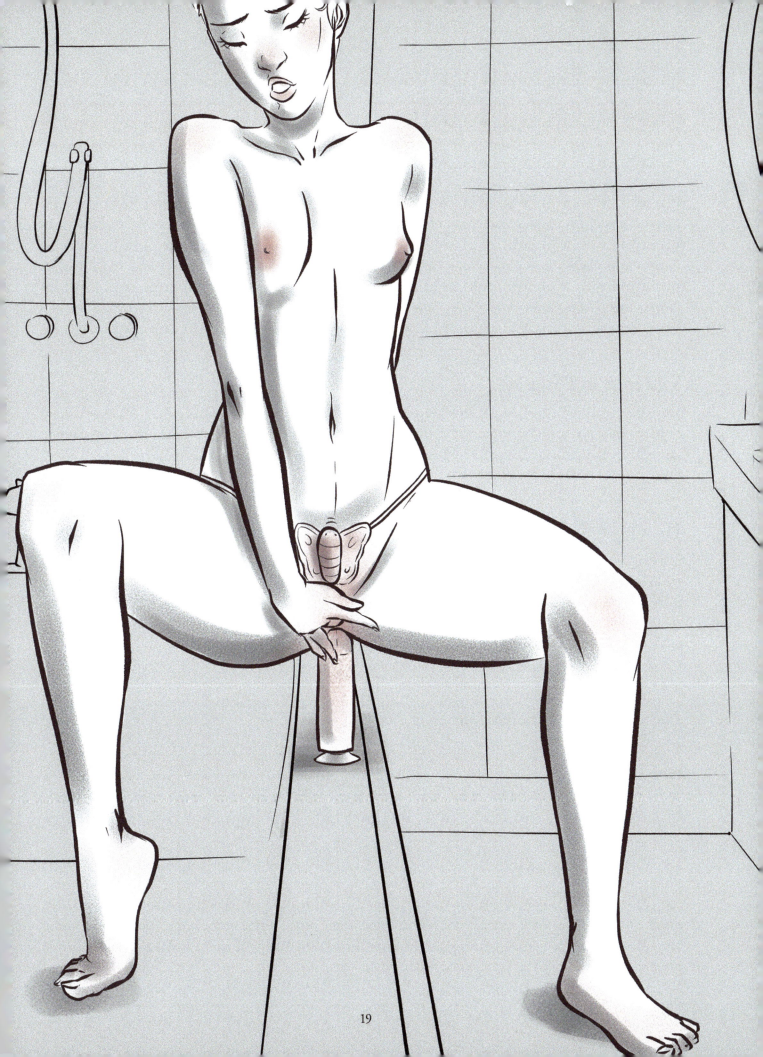

It is imperative that at this point I mention the importance of hygiene at the risk of repeating something you may already know. The adult toy store also sells special lubricants which will not damage the texture of your "tools." Why is this important? Because those "tools" have a non-porous surface and we want to keep them that way, so bacteria do not build up. Porous textures serve as a harbor for bacteria which can cause infections. The adult toy store also sells special soaps to clean and care for your toys.

In general, when it comes to sexual health, it is advisable to ask your gynecologist for guidance on this matter. I was once told that nothing should go into my vagina. . . . Ha! That is a very limiting, short-sighted piece of advice. I did not follow up on that. I hope there are more open-minded gynecologists now who are willing to teach women about self-care and tools maintenance. I can only add to wash your hands before and after with antibacterial soap. Wash your "tools" before and after with special cleaners, and do not put any sugary food in your vagina because the yeast will overpopulate. Most importantly, always remember do not go near the pussy once you have touched the anus. Wash yourself and your toys so that you have a clean start next time.

Vibrators in Disguise

Traveling can throw havoc on our routines and sometimes on our masturbating practices. And I would be embarrassed if my "tools" were exposed in the airline inspection line to the other travelers. I have found some inconspicuous aids that can help. As I mentioned a few pages back, sometimes we must use tools in a way that may have not been intended to satisfy your specific needs.

11. Microdermabrasion

A few years ago, I purchased for the first time a personal microdermabrasion system so I could scrape the old skin cells off my face. As soon as I opened the package, I saw this beautiful tool that vibrates at different speeds; the best part was that the vibrating end was large and round. Oh! My first impression was soon confirmed. As I first tried it on my pussy, the large vibrating head covered much more area than my current vibrator. So now this is one of my favorite vibrators, and I often take it with me when I travel. Yes, I pack the lotions, but just for appearances; I do not exfoliate my face that much.

12. Mechanical Toothbrush

A mechanical toothbrush is also a great asset for the mild-mannered, easy to satisfy pussy. While this is an excellent vibrator in disguise, exercise caution; make sure the vibrating tip is not the kind that slides back and forth creating an opening where your skin can get caught . . . ouch! To be safe, you can cover it with a lubricated (or non-lubricated) condom or a finger cot while in use. Then just throw away the wrap and your toothbrush is still clean.

13. Always Available

The last resort and always available are your fingertips. I am sure many of you have already used your index finger to massage your clit to excite yourselves. Next time, at the point of excitement, bring your other index finger to the entrance of your vagina. Do what pleases you; feel the entrance and tease yourself and or penetrate yourself while you keep rubbing your clit.

The Food Section

This next section is about my favorite foods to aid in my masturbation practices. I am well aware many of you have already been daring and experimented with foods such as honey, mousse, ice cream, cake icing, etc., and rest assured that it makes me proud that you would still take the time to read this book hoping you may learn something new. It would also make me incredibly happy to know that I did not disappoint you.

14. Buttery Delicious

Sometimes the sensual feeling can be brought on by the food that fuels a sweet, comforting feeling within us . . . A lazy Sunday morning while you are still feeling soft and slinky, you notice that butter (unsalted) makes everything taste so much better. After spreading some over your toast, rub some butter on your nipples and add sprinkles of sugar, honey, or anything else that suits your taste. Now taste! If you are not able to taste yourself, do not worry, you can keep massaging and rubbing your nipples. Keep rubbing them with butter (best if it is a stick of butter at room temperature). Notice how your nipples become hard and protrude. Feel… enjoy the sensuous atmosphere created in your mind, and soon your pussy will also crave the attention. Bring the butter stick down to your pussy slightly touching you along the way. Now, pull your lips apart and slowly stroke your clitoris; oh, that soft, creamy feeling is bewitching! At this point, you can follow your specific, individual needs. Should you leave the butter to move on to a vibrator? Should you penetrate yourself with your soft, buttery finger? Or all the above? Whatever you choose to do is the beauty of your unique sensual goddess command. I cannot take credit for this buttery idea. I saw the initial nipple tasting in a movie. However, my imagination took me much further, and the experimentation can be done with other forms of food.

15. Irish Cream

A very popular Irish Cream liqueur is a favorite; a shot glass is a perfect size to dip your nipples and taste while you fondle yourself rubbing that pussy underneath your dress or skirt. A perfect way to start the evening feeling sexy for the rest of the night: take the time to fix your hair and make-up while still naked or semi-dressed in your sexy lingerie. For the rest of the evening, you become *that* beautiful woman, with an aura of sensuality that men can perceive but do not understand. This feeling within allows you to be selective; for a man or woman to meet your standards, the chosen one must meet you at that higher level of spiritual sensuality. You will feel it because your physical needs are completely satisfied beyond the usual requirements. Your senses are heightened and open to perceive the one, the chosen one.

16. The Always Hard Vegetables

If you choose to stay in and explore other pleasure venues, be daring. . . try a cucumber or carrot. The stiffness may be a bit harsh, so I recommend using an effective natural lubricant. Just keep in mind to start fondling, caressing yourself first. Close your eyes and touch yourself on your neck, feel yourself . . . touch your breasts or massage the lowest part of your buttocks with baby oil or oils made for massage. Rubbing your clitoris is always a great primer, but you do not have to. Find out if you like it rough. If your pussy is wet enough just fuck yourself with it. Vegetables are always available. Just make sure that you make up a reasonable explanation as to why that carrot is in the trash.

17. Chinese Eggplant, Hmmmm

A while back I discovered a Chinese eggplant. I was so awed by it that I posted it on my Facebook account: "My mother said vegetables were good for me, but I did not believe her until I ran into this Chinese eggplant." A large squash is also a good stiff vegetable. Remember that vegetables should always be washed, and it is best to use organic (pesticide free). Lubrication is also especially important as some of these vegetables' texture may cause some irritation. The zucchini's texture is not recommendable; the Mexican squash has a smoother texture perfect for penetration without irritating.

18. Chocolate – Serves Many Purposes

Lindt Lindor Chocolate Truffles are my favorite. They remind me of my feminine sensuality, a slightly hard exterior only tough enough to hold the sweetness from pouring out. As I crack one open, I lick the inside and cannot help but to think of my pussy and how it melts as it is licked. I usually proceed to rub my clit, my nipples, and my lips with what is left of the chocolate before I eat it and move to the next one (then I wash the sugar right away to prevent yeast infection).

Other Ways to Love Yourself

19. Plump Pussy Cat and Its Forgotten Orifice

A relaxing siesta was on my mind when I went to my bed on a quiet Saturday afternoon. But as soon as I sat on the edge of my bed, I looked across the room at my image in the closet door mirror. The image of a soft, plump middle-aged woman, with the feeling of a sleek pussy cat purring for attention, and the scent of my new orchids in full bloom all contributed to the waking of my sensual senses. I reached for my latest favorite vibrator, "the bullet," and gently began to masturbate, tilting back just a tad, while holding the bullet right under my clit, over the entrance to my pleasure tunnel, still looking at myself in the mirror. Surely you think this is something I already mentioned, but wait! Let me finish before you make up your mind about this method.

After a while, feeling so wet and hungry for more sensations, I fully rest my back on the bed and raise my legs still spread apart, keeping my knees bent with the soles of my feet pointing to the ceiling. Still feeling the bullet's pulsating vibrations that compound my excitement, I take my index finger (yes, I mentioned this before, but wait). I take my index finger and with its very tip, I feel the orifice of my pussy. I am not penetrating, I am exploring, feeling, getting to know that very small part of me that can play a huge role in my sexual satisfaction. As you do this, you will feel your body heat up; you will feel the waves of pleasure erupting from that ridiculously small, hardly explored, often underestimated part of your pussy. After I did it for the first time, I was laughing, bursting with joy. The satisfaction was so unique and exhilarating.

If you do this without the vibrator stimulation on your clit, it will take longer, and you may not reach the ecstasy I am describing. The vibrator rapidly takes you to the point of excitation necessary for this phenomenal experience. The reason being that this part of your pussy is always taken for granted. This part of you is seen merely as a path to the goal. What we have failed to see is that the whole pussy is filled with nerves and this part, the very entrance to our mystical pussy, is the most sensitive part, second only to your clit.

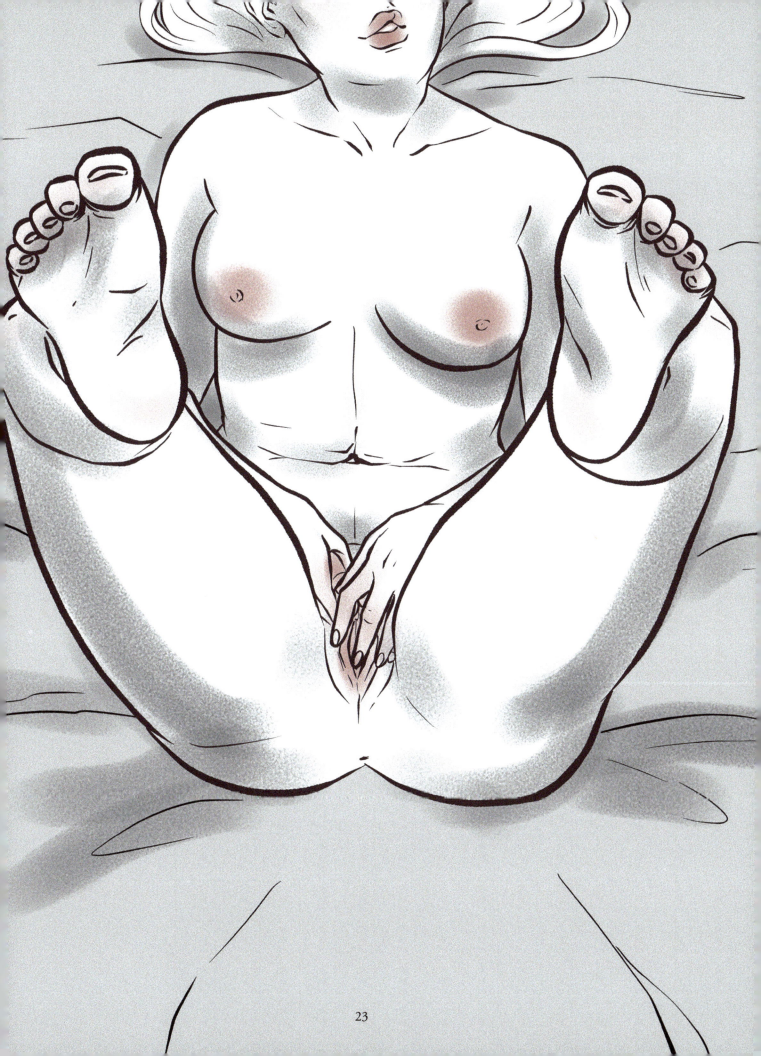

20. Go Fuck Yourself. . . . And Smile

In a very daring moment, I surprised myself; it was an extremely hot summer afternoon when I arrived home and quickly undressed to get over the heat overcoming my body. As I felt the cool air on my skin, my senses reawakened and my nipples hardened as I saw myself in the mirror. I could not help but reach for the usual . . . vibrator and dildo. I soon succumbed to the awesome feeling of ecstasy but not quite to orgasm. Watching myself and my eager pussy swallowing that dildo, I was feeling so good, but I sensed this time I needed more. I pulled out my anal probe, turned around at the edge of my bed and kept the vibrator between my pussy lips while the dildo remained in my pussy. I slowly took the probe and buried it in my ass, while I looked back to the mirror as I fucked myself. The view was so hot, just like those hot, super sexy women on pornographic videos. So now when someone tells you "go fuck yourself," just grin and remember how good it will feel when you do.

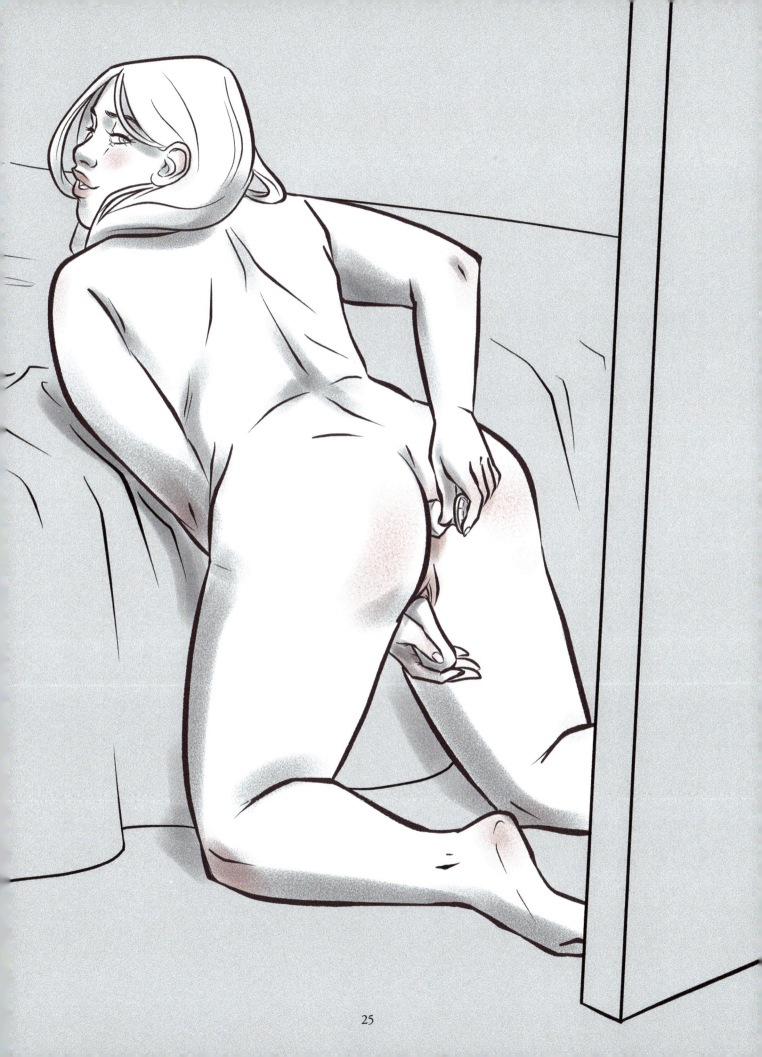

21. Forceful Penetration (no, I do not mean unwelcome penetration)

Lastly, when you crave to feel the forceful penetration of hard cock, try it with your pajamas on. Usually when I do this, I begin with just my hand over my pussy circulating, feeling it; it almost takes an identity of its own. Soon I proceed with the bullet vibrator because I can place it between my pussy lips, and it will stay put while still sending those awesome vibrations. Then, when I get really hot and my pussy is so wet with its natural, musky potion, I take the hardest dildo (pajamas are still on) and place it between the crotch of my pajamas and the orifice of my pussy. By keeping your pajamas in place, you are creating a force pushing the dildo into your pussy. If necessary, you can also pull your pajamas (at your discretion) to accentuate the forceful dildo fucking you. Do not immediately push your dildo; tease your pussy; accentuate that feeling of being penetrated, forcefully penetrated. Ohhhh! What a feeling!

Note: Please take note that when I say forceful penetration, I envision a big cock pushing his way into a hot and willing yet tight pussy. I HAVE NO INTENTION TO INSINUATE UNWANTED INTERCOURSE.

I am a strong believer in consensual sex; this book is fueled by that belief because women do like to fuck. If a man must force, coerce, drug, intimidate, etc., a woman to have sex with him, then he is completely, unequivocally, and criminally wrong.

22. Find a Way to Love Yourself

Loving ourselves does not always involve sexual acts. Time for pampering is important, although many of us let that go when we have others to take care of, such as small children, elderly parents, sick spouses, etc. It is only natural to fully dedicate ourselves to the ones we love. However, pampering is another way we love ourselves. A short, simple routine can make a huge difference in our well-being. Every morning I take some cool moisturizing eye drops and a Ziploc baggie half full of water from the fridge. I lay down on my couch where I have placed my foot massager. I turn on the massager and I put the cool soothing eye drops in my eyes and place the baggie over them. I have learned to relax for the term of my massage; about 15 to 30 minutes. It is a wonderful feeling; I feel loved. It is important that you find that routine; it may take time, but try to picture yourself where you feel loved. I, for some strange reason, feel mostly loved resting on the branch of a huge tree. I believe it is the feeling of living with the strong support that you feel from something more than a father or mother. I have always loved trees and climbed them often when I was a child. The strength of a tree that supported me and my swings was an unforgettable feeling.

23. Start Treating Yourself with Love

Most important is to love yourself by treating yourself right and putting a bit of a distance between you and the negative people around you. You know who…the friends, acquaintances, and relatives whom you try to avoid but somehow you give in because they need someone to talk to. However, their venting of problems is never-ending, and it seems to increase as they see your sincere attempt to comfort them. They will only take your time and sour your outlook. Love yourself by not allowing them to suck your positive energy. Life is too short to spend it with people who live to complain—in doing so they miss all the beauty, all the wonderfulness around us.

SECTION III
Flying with Your Lover

It took time for me to begin this section. I was unsure of how to express the need to love yourself and how it can be done while loving your partner. I strongly believe that the love for yourself should be incorporated in your lovemaking; this is the only path to true satisfaction.

Unaware in my younger years, I now see that the ultimate level of your sexuality is to feel so comfortable with your partner and it feels so natural, that loving yourself becomes a part of your lovemaking. This is no easy task; it is more like a journey on which couples embark without a compass or any kind of guidance.

But how can we reach that level of intimacy, you may ask? Or, what level of intimacy am I referring to? This level of intimacy takes some time to build; it cannot be reached overnight regardless of your sexual prowess. Once your partner has seen you in your worst moments and he/she still stands by you, supporting you and loving you… when you feel that your partner is committed to you by their own will and speak of being together in the future even though neither of you is sure what that future will be… when your partner lovingly acknowledges but looks past your imperfections . . . *then* you are at the ideal point in a relationship where both of you can reach that level of intimacy.

Another major factor that deserves our attention is the energy emitting from within us and from our lovers. We all have that energy emitting from our psychic core. Some of us are overly sensitive to that energy, while others are not; however, we all share that spiritual essence and we all can sense it. If your energy is filled with resentment, doubt, nervousness, or shame about your partner, about the sexual moment, or about your sexuality, then your partner will feel it and more than likely accept it as his/her feelings. The following experience is a perfect example of the conflicting energies that cause so much confusion in our sensual world.

I met Arnold one hot summer on one of those online dating sites. Soon we were communicating mostly through poetry, our thoughts and feelings leading to our unique writing. We seemed to click mystically; so much so that by the second time we met in person, we were intimate. Quickly I learned that Arnold emitted such strong energy that it would almost paralyze me. And even though he was a master in massaging me to ecstasy, I found myself behaving awkwardly. I was not confident enough to allow my full sensual, sexual self free. I felt like a deer in front of the blinding headlights, in awe of the beauty of the light but frozen. Thus, every time we had sex, I became the receiver.

Only after some distance, I realized that I was not at ease for other reasons besides Arnold's strong presence. Our sexual encounters did not add too much to the relationship. He had not seen me at my worst moments and stayed by my side; he certainly was not committed to nurturing a romantic relationship with me; my imperfections did not seem to bother him but he was not at all taken by my looks or any other qualities. So even though our "sexual chemistry" sizzled, the actual act of loving ourselves was as fluid as Dwayne Johnson dancing tango in the movie *Red Notice (2021)*. How could I have shown him the real me when I did not feel fully accepted as a loving partner?

This is the heart of the issue when trying to love yourself and your partner: to feel fully accepted, to feel beautiful inside and out. In all my sexual relationships, this feeling was achieved with only one lover. But most important was the realization that marriage does not guarantee this loving acceptance. Sure, we talk about it and we think we have achieved it; however, you do not know chocolate until you have tasted it. And once you have tasted real chocolate, you can quickly identify the watered-down versions.

Before Arnold, there was Erick, the love of my life. I worked with Erick for a year before we started to date. I soon learned he was a highly skilled lover, but what made him so great was his ability to make me feel beautiful, insatiable; the more he tasted, the more he wanted. I had never experienced this eagerness, this drive, this desire for me. The most effective aphrodisiac is to feel so desired; but most importantly, he also made me feel accepted.

One such occasion was on my birthday. He was coming to pick me up for a night out. As I was taking a bath, I made the mistake to leave my hearing aids on the side of my tub, which was also within the reach of my dog. She chewed those things up in seconds. I was devastated; I texted him about canceling. He came by anyway and comforted me. I was in tears; however, he managed to make that night a beautiful experience. We did not go anywhere; he brought dinner and a couple of movies to watch. He was so sweet making up some sign language of his own and just being there for me, holding me.

It is moments like these that build up intimacy. These are the moments that build confidence in our relationship and for us to fully express our sexuality. The spiritual freedom I felt after living so many moments such as these with him gave me the courage to explore further. I had the courage to show him how I masturbate. I even dared to express and explore my bisexuality; we joined a swingers' website and met with some lovely couples on occasion.

It took me 45 years to find this level of intimacy. I probably would have reached it before in previous relationships, but neither I nor my partners were wise enough. I hope that this book helps people realize that the treasure lies in our relationships, and I hope that they strive to nurture these relationships before they reach middle age. In these electronic dating times, it is easy to get lost in the vast amount of superficial connections with potential lovers. The danger is to quickly move on to the next one because we are looking for a 100% compatible human being. This ideal will never be fulfilled because, even if we find someone so compatible, the feelings of trust, candidness, and love take time to develop. The lack of wisdom to be patient and allow them the time is our tragic mistake; in essence, we have become disposable partners.

Also, please take note that our sexuality is a different universe, as unique as our DNA; therefore, do not assume that exploring your sexuality will drive you to "become" bisexual, homosexual, etc.

Encourage your lover, but do not expect them to feel at ease with threesomes or orgies. Expectations have a way of hampering any special bonding moments. If it is something that exists within your lover, it will float to the surface, and it will have a drive of its own. It is much more beautiful when the woman feels confident enough in the commitment, in her beauty, and in the relationship that she initiates experimentation. Also, note that the most beautiful gesture is for someone to want to know you; and the more you know your lover, the better lover you will be to him or her. Moreover, as you read these "techniques," keep in mind that there has been plenty of mental and sexual foreplay, lots of kissing and caressing, and plenty of tenderness and caring affirmations.

It has been my experience that most men love to see a woman take pleasure in herself, and smart men know that her sex toys can save them some time and effort. A smart lover makes a woman come many times before he/she penetrates her. Why? Because as mentioned earlier, a woman can come so many times and keep going while a man's erections are limited. So, men, use your energy and her toys wisely.

Gentlemen and bi ladies, it is highly recommendable that your hands are well-groomed because your fingers will get the call for pussy duty, and a manicure is preferred. Jagged fingernails and old skin around the cuticle can hurt the pussy. If you want to be nice to her, use one of those face scrubs to massage your hands before you wash them. The scrub will take away so much of the dead skin leaving you with soft and smooth fingers. You can also use sugar with coconut oil to create a scrubbing paste. Massage your hands and fingers and around the fingernails well before you rinse in warm water. After you wash your hands, you may not feel the need for hand lotion because of the coconut oil but still put some on to protect your baby soft hands; after a scrub, your skin is open and will take the nourishment of the hand lotion. Your hands will get so much softer when you practice this often. Your hands will be soft and gentle, perfect for pussy penetration.

24. It Is Ok to Take the Lead

I have taken the lead on some occasions by using my vibrator while my partner is fetching us more wine or the massage oils. In just minutes, I am purring like a cat and eager for my partner to fondle me. As he steps back into the room, he gets an immediate hard-on (if he did not already have one), and he pounces on me like a tiger eager to devour its catch. I keep the slow, smooth vibrations going while my partner caresses me, kisses me. At this point, there are several different ways to go.

25. Warming Up with Mr. V

While you still have your vibrator near or on your clit, your partner can insert his finger into your vagina gently, slowly, and no more than two inches. Slowly work the finger in and out while kissing her or nibbling on her nipples. This activity usually makes the woman come but just enough to serve as a warmup. When my partner does this, I soon squirm, screaming "fuck me" because it wakes up the insatiable pussy.

26. He Licks Because He Likes It

Oh, but a smart lover does not go straight to fucking yet. He will go down and continue working on that pussy. No more vibrator; now comes the wet, luscious, very skilled tongue. It will take a while to come again; while he licks so slowly and lovingly, you sense that he licks because he likes it. A surge of "I am beautiful" travels from your pussy to your brain and to your whole being. At this point, loving you means accept it. Accept that feeling and do whatever comes to you. Talk the dirtiest talk you have ever imagined, or just scream how beautiful you feel. Whatever you do will be ok, I assure you. Pull his hair (but not too hard), scratch his back, etc., just do not hurt him unless he is okay with that.

27. More Fingers, More PC Muscle Contractions

Soon you will start moaning and humming; floating again in ecstasy; when he senses that you are ready, he again, brings in his hand and inserts two fingers. Why two? Because you are ready for more. Ladies, at this point, it is time to exercise your PC muscle. For me, it is second nature, but in the beginning, we must remind ourselves. The PC muscle helps you feel so much more. The "in and out" thrust of the fingers coupled with your pussy squeezing them will soon have you humming and moaning.

It is important to note that if the pussy is being licked out of obligation, it will be noticed and will affect the outcome. As mentioned earlier, the energy we emit communicates our true selves; thus, your lover will know, and the moment will be hindered. Communication/feedback is imperative, and the more you communicate the better your lover and you will be to each other. For example, are you ok with two fingers? Maybe you are ready for three. While your lover fingers you, what else would you like him to do?

28. Add to the Activity

It is ok to add to the activity—meaning that while pussy licking and probing is going on, you can contribute to and build on the experience. Feel yourself. Get to know the feel of your skin, the feel of your nipples at your most excited state. You will soon learn what your body wants and it will depend on what you prefer; I can only give you an example of what I do because our sexuality is so unique.

Experimenting is your best option to find what you and your lover get off to. I prefer that he gently bites my nipples. Early on in our sexual sessions, I began to massage my breasts while he was fingering me and was so hot that I started licking, then sucking on my breasts. He saw me doing that, so he started doing it while still fingering me, never missing a beat. When I started to come, I screamed "bite me," and he immediately complied. Now he knows that I come even stronger when he (gently) bites my nipples, and it makes me squirt at times. He also knows that timing is important. You must communicate that as well. The moment I reach orgasm is the right time for me. The bite needs to start soft until you both find out how hard of a bite you can take.

Remember that communication is also the loving kisses that we give each other while teasing and pleasing ourselves. Your lover can finger you and still kiss you so romantically, or ferociously. The important thing is to develop communication between you that continues through your lovemaking. Our lover must know he is on the right track to pleasure. We all need feedback. We want to know if what we are doing is effective or not, if it is fucking hot or you could be fine without it.

At this point you may be asking, how am I loving myself while with a partner? Yes, he is doing all the lovemaking but by…

29. Squeeze Your PC

…squeezing your PC muscle, you are masturbating while your partner is kissing you and fingering you. As you squeeze, your sensations are multiplied and you are warming up. There is a build-up of excitement that you are nurturing, which will carry you to a higher level of ecstasy.

30. Suck, Lick, Bite Yourself

By sucking, licking, and biting your nipples, you are loving your body as well. Again, this comes easier to those who are very comfortable with their bodies but, even if you are not quite there, pretend that you are, and soon it will be second nature to love your body as you are being loved by your lover.

31. Accept the Feeling

Accepting that awesome feeling of being loved, appreciated, and desired is loving yourself. This is a concept that many of us underestimate and sometimes difficult to achieve if we are weighted down with so many insecurities or traumas. It may take some time to learn to accept that you are one hot pussy who deserves to be devoured, to be fucked, and to enjoy it, to be valued, and to be treated with care. I know it sounds like a cliché, but repeating loving affirmations that remind you that you deserve to be loved may help. You could even make it a foreplay game with your lover. If you have the one you love to repeat to you in a hot, sexy voice: "You deserve to be loved; your pussy deserves to be licked like it's the best ice cream ever made; you deserve to be fucked till your eyes roll back with overwhelming pleasure; you deserve me to make love to you." The wording may be changed to suit your taste. Some people do not like explicit language, and it may make them more uncomfortable.

Some of us may have deep-rooted issues that need counseling, time, and patience. This is your call, but do not leave this matter unattended. It is more important than you realize.

32. I Ride, I Command

Let us backtrack a bit. During our teenage years, we likely became masters at masturbating by rubbing against each other so that we could obtain some satisfaction while sex was still out of the question. But why stop such activity just because we have "grown up"? I have also done this with some dates on occasions, long after my teenage years. The reasons varied, but I found it to be playful. To improve the sensations, wear loose and thin clothing, climb onto him so you can have control of your movements, and keep kissing him as you rub against his cock. For example, after a movie, my date and I came back to my house for a drink. It had not been long since I had first met him and still did not feel sure about his intentions. Somehow, I felt that he was just after sexual relations for which I was not interested. I was looking for a committed relationship. We were sitting on the couch enjoying some wine and conversation when I brought one leg over him which positioned me sitting on his lap, facing him fully clothed. We started kissing and I got hot, so I started rubbing my pussy against his hard cock. I did an excellent job of bringing myself to orgasm. It is important to note that this procedure is achieved with greater satisfaction if your clothes are very thin and not hampering your lively pussy with tight pantyhose or jeans. For example, I was not wearing panties and my outfit was a thin cotton jumper.

And now, my personal favorites of loving myself while with my partner; riding high has been my favorite position since I became a self-confident, determined lover. This position gives me so much control over what I want to get out of fucking, but yet it can also be so romantic.

33. Lay and Stay, I Say

While feeling playful and wanting to conserve my lover's energy, I instruct him to just lay and stay. I climb on his cock but do not take him in entirely. I squat and lower myself only far enough to allow his head to come in. I go up and down feeling his bulbous head force its way in expecting to be completely swallowed by my eager pussy, but no, only the head until I say so. My pussy tightens as it gets excited, and it is not long before I get so hot that I take in more. It takes strong legs to do this. It also helps to have something to hold onto so that your arms can help you ease the weight from your legs. Because this is so awesome, I am considering placing some handles on the wall above my headboard. I know there will be questions about them, and I'm not sure how to answer them. The handles would help me hold on so that I can last longer than my legs allow.

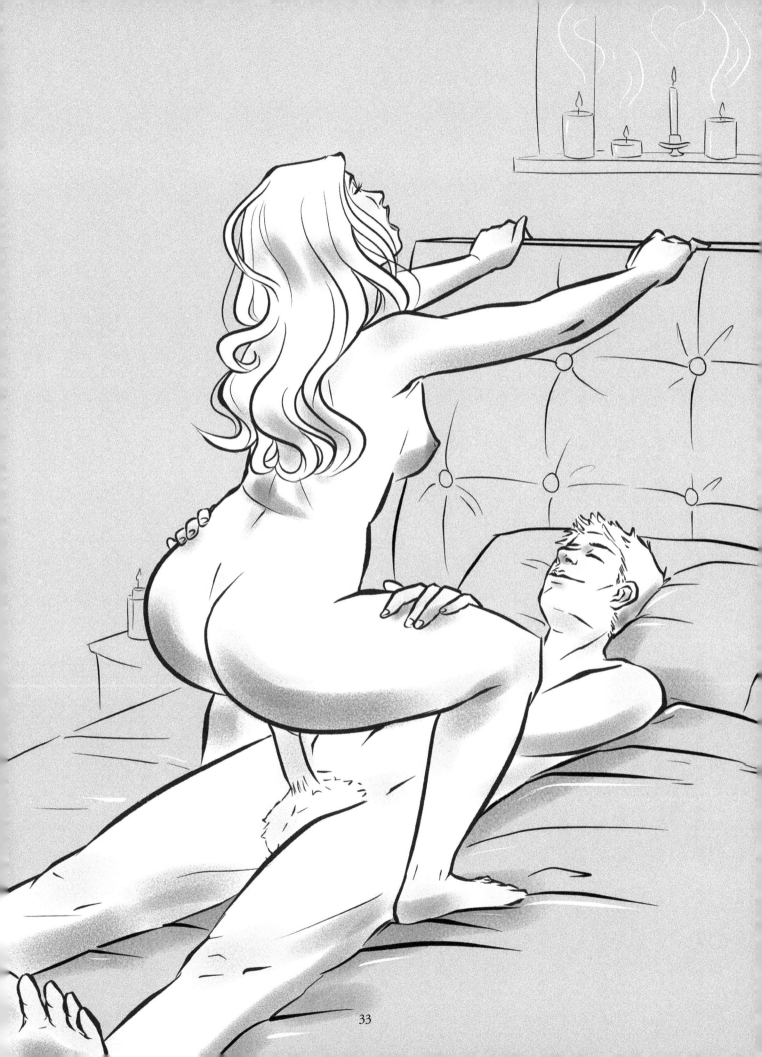

34. Bring in the Reinforcements – Mr. V

On another occasion, or the same lovemaking session, when my legs tire of squatting, I let my pussy swallow that cock and rest my weight on him; I then take my vibrator and start the vibrations on my clit. Again, I tell him to not move. Men tend to think that their movement will help but, on this occasion, his movement will delay my excitement. Let the vibrator do the work. My pussy starts getting hot again. Feeling the vibrations deep inside my pussy now stuffed with cock, I can feel the wetness, sticky humid wetness, which is quickly followed by my contractions. At this point, my lover is now so excited feeling squeezed and wet. I get so hot I cannot help but to scream in ecstasy. This is extremely exciting for both of us; soon it is overwhelming, and I stop the vibrator and my lover takes over. It is his turn to fuck me with all his might.

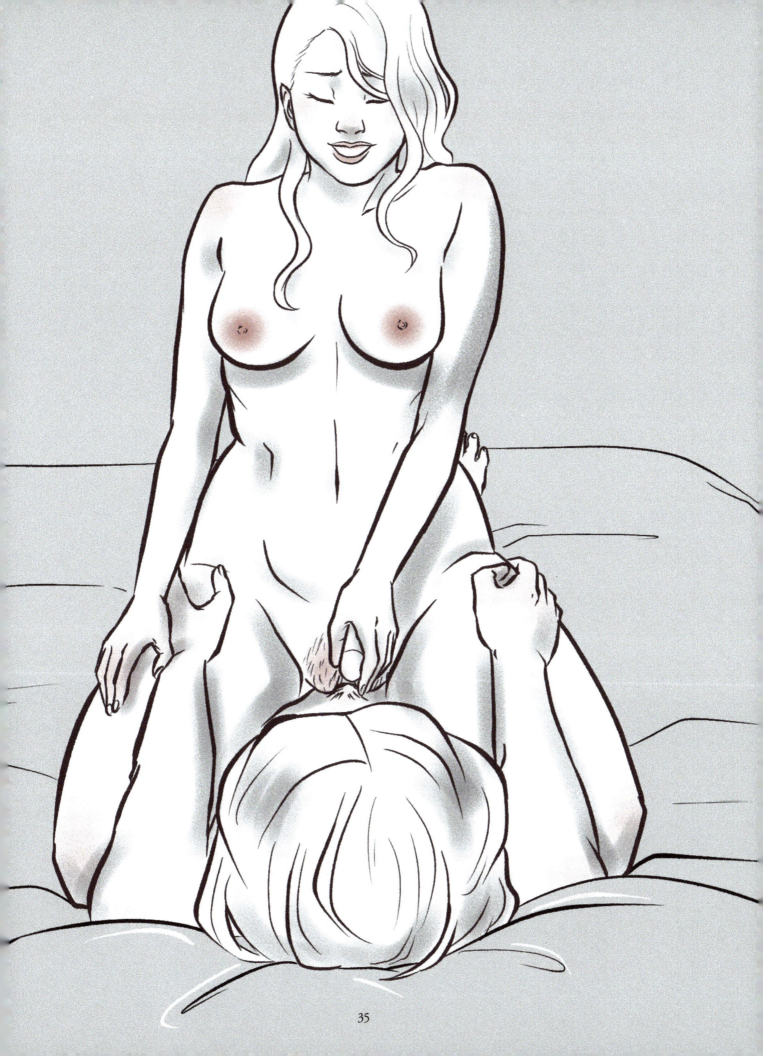

35. Bite Me . . . or Whatever You Prefer

While still on #34 and the vibrator is working its magic; feeling pure ecstasy flowing from your pussy up to your whole body, before he takes over, ask him to gently bite your nipples, to clasp his teeth on your neck and/or your shoulder muscles. You may find this will elevate you even higher.

36. Locked and Loaded Sex Rock

Number 34 with a clasp made with my legs around him while he is sitting straight up. This can be done on the bed or the couch. I place my hands on the headboard or the back of the couch and lock my arms to create a tense hold while I only move my hips back and forth. This thrusting motion accentuates the PC and glutes muscles and works them to exhilarating exhaustion. This position serves to masturbate myself while fucking him and getting the best workout for a sexy body, all at the same time.

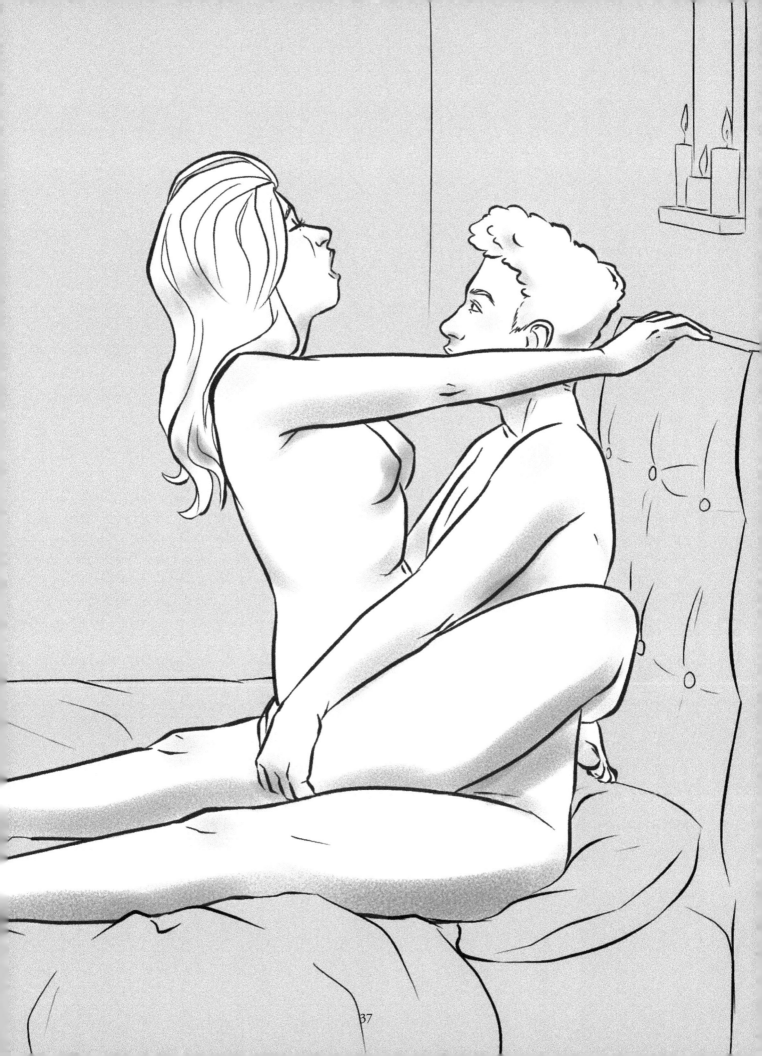

37. No. 34 Reversed with Butt Plug

Number 34 reversed and at the point of ecstasy still holding the vibrator on my clit, I yell "fuck me." That is the signal. That is when my lover knows I am ready and, as previously instructed, reaches for the dildo, and plunges it into my ass when I bend forward (toward his toes). He then plunges it in and out at a moderate speed. You must tell him what "moderate" means to you because he will not know, and we all have specific preferences. Remember, communication is the key.

38. Shower Poke and Swallow

When I found a wall with a handle, I rejoiced. That wall was the shower at my boyfriend's house. This was an old shower with the old tile and the towel bar also of ceramic tile. We often took showers with him back to the wall and me placing my feet on the edges of the tub, facing him, and holding on to that towel bar. Oh, I rocked (literally). I was able to tease him and myself by just letting his head (penis) poke inside my pussy. I would randomly swallow him completely and always squeezed him with my pussy (PC muscle).

39. Jane (from Tarzan) and the Towel Bar

On other occasions, I would do all the above mentioned. Head first, then full cock with a waterproof vibrator. The same principle, he would just stand firm like a little soldier saluting me with his hard cock. I was like Jane (from Tarzan) holding on to the towel bar with the left hand, holding my vibrator with my right, and pressing it on my clit while my pussy swallowed his head. As my excitement increased my pussy would swing, fucking him more, and more. Once I reached my orgasm, which was unmistakable because I am screaming in ecstasy and my pussy is contracting to squeeze him so tight, I let go of the vibrator and he would grab me by the hips to rock me back and forth till we both came. Yes, I was in a continuous orgasmic phase.

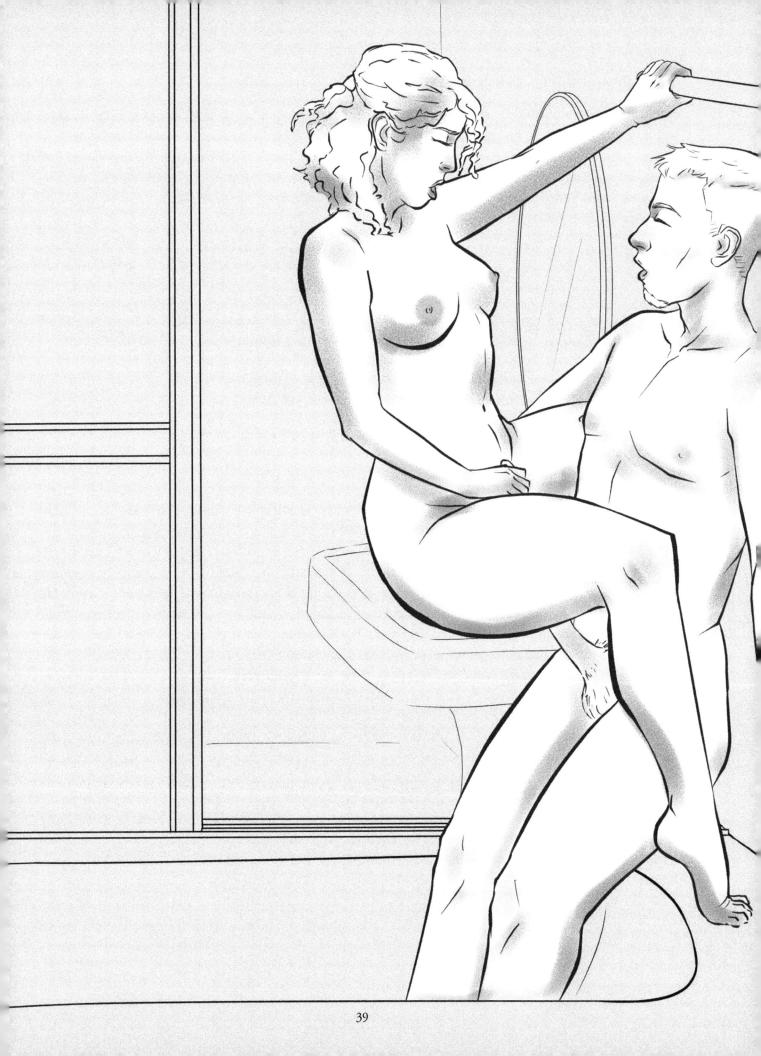

40. Jane and the Confident Lover

Finally, as I mentioned before, sometimes you just need more than a pussy fuck, you need it in the ass. I had my dildo ready in the shower, and at the peak of ecstasy, I asked him to use the dildo. He was always so happy to comply with double fucking with the dildo in my ass. This is very pleasurable for the man as well because of the extra pressure placed within the vagina. So, by pleasuring yourself, he also gets his pleasure maximized. Ask and you shall receive . . . this is mostly true when making love with a confident lover. You are loving yourself when you ask for what pleases you.

There is something particularly important to be cognizant of. While each of these ways of loving yourself is listed and numbered may seem so mechanical, they are not. There are plenty of kisses, caresses, and loving affirmations before, during, and after. At first, we may act a bit clumsy; this is like when you begin dance lessons. You are trying to remember the right sequence of steps to follow and thus you cannot enjoy a relaxed conversation. However, as time passes, you will get into your natural flow, your natural rhythm.

I grew up with few choices. I do not blame anyone; it was due partly to our poverty and partly to our culture. Early in life, I learned that imagination could provide you with the choices you naturally crave and deserve. Allow for that imagination to lead you to the world you want to create. You will be much happier.

41. Accountants are Underestimated Sexual Machines

Your imagination is another sex toy, even better than vibrators and dildos. The two kinkiest lovers I have been with are accountants. Interestingly, they both loved storytelling. I was taught by the first accountant, and I blossomed as a storyteller with the second accountant. The first one was expressive of what he wanted from me, but I was young and insecure. I learned from that experience, and when I was with Accountant #2 (about 15 years later) I noticed that just a simple sexual act was not enough for him to reach orgasm. He needed more stimulation, but my mouth was tired of sucking his cock, so I started talking to him. I put some massage oil on my hand and started my hand-job while telling him a story of office sex. I noticed that he was immediately captivated, and his cock felt like it was going to explode in my hand…his skin was so tight, and his penis grew larger than I had ever seen it before. My stories grew in complexity and with more vivid descriptions.

There is a downside to this practice. Your lover needs to fully trust you and to differentiate truth from storytelling. Accountant #2 grew suspicious, thinking that I had participated in at least some of the stories, if not all. Our relationship suffered because he felt that I did not want to introduce him to those people (the characters in my stories). Trust, communication, acceptance, and respect are the keys to keeping a sexual practice like the above mentioned; without those elements, a relationship will sour and eventually will tear down any loving feelings that had brought you together in the first place. Even if I had participated in those stories, my lover should have accepted that I did not want to engage again with him involved. The respect that the past is past and the present is open and mutually enjoyable is essential.

42. Mobile Butterfly

On my way to a sexual encounter, I was happily trying out the new additions to my collection— the nipple grippers and the "G-spot butterfly" vibrator. The butterfly has straps that hold it in place, so I was able to walk about freely to and from my car. My blouse was layered with ruffles so that the nipple grippers were not noticeable. So, armed and sexy, I hopped in my car to my rendezvous. I reached minor orgasms a couple of times before I made it to my destination, but that did not put a damper on my evening. Upon arrival, my friend discovered what I was doing, and he was immediately excited. He fucked and fucked and fucked me as I was still excited. You see, my minor orgasms were but mere warmups that only opened me up for a much higher experience with my partner. About an hour later, we went to dinner and hurried back to fuck some more.

43. Riding the Bullet

On another occasion, my blouse was elegantly layered so that I could rest the bullet wire and control in the layered pocket while the bullet was in between my pussy lips. My nipple clips were gently but firmly gripped to my nipples, this time with tiny weights to heighten the stimulation. I drove to my friend's fantasizing about being stopped by a policeman. Unfortunately, I am an exceptionally good driver, so my fantasy did not realize. I enjoyed the drive with a "Mona Lisa smile" all the way. This time I set the control for very mild vibrations to just excite my pussy without reaching orgasm. The drive was exhilarating. When I got to my friend's I was so ready to fuck.

44. Ask and You Shall Receive

An example of "ask and you shall receive" happened to me on a date that ended up on my couch. All the kissing and hugging led to the fondling, which led to some extremely exciting, half-disrobing, pussy probing by my incredibly talented partner. He never missed a beat kissing me, gently rubbing my pussy with his tongue. I was incredibly pleased; however, that was not enough for me. I took his index finger and brought it to my vagina and softly whispered "fuck me." He complied again without missing a beat, without stopping the super sexy tongue stimulation he was giving me. I was even more excited. He kept going and noticed that I was exhilarated but seemed to need more (he later told me). So, he gave me more; without stopping, he inserted the rest of his fingers into my ass and I am so lucky he did. I was flying high; I felt as though I was soaring up in the sky, weightless and beautiful. I felt so good that I remember screaming "this is so fucking beautiful."

I believe this is the first time he learned to eat pussy while finger fucking it. I was fortunate to be with a loving partner who sincerely wanted to please me; he was a true, unselfish lover. But even the most wonderful lover needs to know what his or her partner needs. And, the only way is to communicate your wish, your desire, to your lover. This is another way of loving yourself; ask for what you want and need.

Note: I did not immediately ask for his finger to come into my pussy. I usually reserve this for after some heavy tongue action, and when I have reached a level of excitement that will be attained with the tongue alone. I believe this is enough stimulation for some, but for the more experienced and vigorous lovers, the additional inspirational probing is needed to reach a higher level of ecstasy.

45. A Lover with Penis Control

Another instance of pussy probing to excite was learned from a lover who had amazing control of his penis. He could be so firm and bring it to my pussy without penetration. I could feel the head of his cock just circle the entrance to my eager pussy. As I mentioned earlier, the incredibly soft area at the opening of your vagina is the second most sensitive area of your pussy, but it is often unappreciated and always overlooked.

So how did I turn this into loving myself? I do not expect every male to have this kind of control over his cock, so I take the initiative; I have on occasion taken my partner's erect penis and just rubbed that part of my pussy. I take what I want and do what I want because I love myself. A loving partner will surely be eager to please you.

46. Learn Your True Sexuality – Accept It and Embrace It

Important and inevitable choices (and we should be able to choose) are our lover(s), our lifestyle, and our openness—they all impact our sexual lives. But the one fact of which we have no choice is that we are sensual beings and we need sexual relations. This is our essence, whether we are heterosexual, homosexual, or bisexual, etc.; we are "wired" this way. We cannot change that. Therefore, it is in our best interest to learn our sexuality, accept it, and embrace it, because in doing so we are loving ourselves.

Note: When I use the term "lifestyle" I am not referring to the terms of bisexuality, homosexuality, etc. I do not consider that to be a lifestyle. Our sexuality is not a choice. It is the essence of our being. Lifestyle means (to me) a choice of how we carry ourselves in this life. My lifestyle, for example, is private in general. I am open to very few people. I am not good with small talk and mostly listen to conversations unless the topic is of great importance and I know the people participating. I do not socialize much but keep connected by meeting friends every two or three months.

We have the choice to make love to ourselves and fully satisfy our sexual need by ourselves, with our partner, with whomever we please.

As a real introvert, I have always been quiet about my opinions and life experiences. Still, we all need to express ourselves, and I am no different—no matter how much of an introvert I claim to be. The great poets and writers, artists of all kinds show the world who they are through their works. This book is my venue to express the need for a better understanding of our amazing female sexuality. When the movie *50 Shades of Grey* came to theaters in every city of America, there was a huge fuss. I found the story to be just that, a story, fiction -with the classical sexual dominant male and far removed from what women genuinely want.

The point is to find the one partner who not only allows you to express yourself but also has an honest interest in what you are expressing as well as trying to deeply understand what you have to say, what you think, and your take on events that affect our lives.

The most important aspect to consider when making love to yourself while loving your partner is to remember the times before he came into your life. Remember not to be sad but to rejoice and take in his scent; allow it to guide you to the universe where only you (both) exist. It has been a while since I have had a "loving partner," and I can attest that without the love, support, and playful acceptance of each other, nothing else can be fulfilling. Love yourself by making sure that your "loving partner" respects you and the essential needs you crave, whether it's a committed relationship, comforting and loving gestures, or even financial restraint to others so he can splurge with you. Again, the only way he will know your essential needs is by you communicating them. When a loving partner wants to engage in acts that we are not in agreement with, it all comes down to one question: "Can I live with this?" Sometimes the search for the answer to this question can lead to a remarkably difficult decision. Whatever you decide is the answer to this self-inquiry: do you love your partner more than yourself?

About my statement above, "without the love, support, and playful acceptance of each other, nothing else can be fulfilling," there is the other side of the spectrum of our free sexual spirits. At times we may find the truest of love with a wonderful partner, but our sexual needs may go unattended. I am sure many have stood at the abyss of mysterious sexuality that we so desire to explore, yet we hold back for various reasons. Our sexuality is powerful, but I still believe that (leaving the sex addicts and criminal sexual deviants aside) on its own is not enough to break a relationship.

SECTION IV
Flying with the crew of your choice

This part of My Pussy's User Manual is more difficult to explain, as it involves anything or anybody outside of the traditional heterosexual couple. With time, we evolve in every aspect including our sexual being. It is healthy to evolve; it is a result of experimentation and self-analysis which is a sign that we are living organisms with the capability of mind development. We are not just amoebas seeking the survival of the species.

47.   Allow for Experimentation and Evolvement

Sometime in the past, I read that "sex begins in the mind."[38] I wholeheartedly agree. So how do I tie in the part of loving yourself to this topic? You love yourself when you allow yourself to explore, to experiment, to fantasize, and try to make those fantasies a reality if that is what you wish. I believe most of us want to do all these things that we dream of, but a concern for our safety holds us back. This encompasses more than physical safety. Our valiant actions depend on our strength of character. The stronger we are, the more willing we are to take a chance as we might expose a deep erotic part of ourselves which others may not understand. This is so true as I have vacillated in making the final decision to publish this book. I know that much of my self will be exposed, and critics will come crawling out of the woodwork like cockroaches seeking to feed on my exposed character. But there is a higher need to express myself than to live in fear of those critics.

48.   Be True to Yourself

Around the age of 45 is when I said "fuck it"—I am what I am and will go where my heart, my mind, and my pussy lead me. This was not an easy step to take; it was immensely helpful to have a supporting partner, which at the time I did. I let my mind go, and scenes started playing in my head like XXX rated movies. My stories/fantasies kept getting more sophisticated to the point I wanted to make them a reality. At this point, I would like to negate the fear of going too far; as you use your judgment without the influence of alcohol and other chemical substances, you will know how much you can take, how far you can go. In a safe sexual environment, you can always say "stop," "enough," "I don't want to do that," or simply walk away. Safety has always been a concern and my top requirement.

The beginning of my experimentation beyond myself and my boyfriend was joining the swingers community. I initiated it. It makes a difference when the woman is the one who initiates and moves forward to accepting others in a sexual scene. My experiences were all wonderful. We met some fabulous couples who were respectful and very tender. Do keep in mind that they are not your friends. Friendships may develop, but

I find that difficult to take place. I came into the swingers' scene aware of that, and a friend re-emphasized this belief. She once confided that she did not care to join any swingers anymore due to her bad experience. She had gone on a swingers' cruise, and it was wonderful fun full of sexual encounters. However, when they returned, she had car problems and not one of the people she had fucked during the cruise stopped to help her or tried to find her help. I view the swingers community like drinking buddies; they will be fun for the moment and you will have a good time, but after that, you are on your own. It will be awesome if good friendships develop, but do not expect it.

The positive aspect of swingers is the loyalty they feel and exhibit toward their partners and the respect they demonstrate toward others and their relationships. I cannot speak for everyone, but my take on this lifestyle is a sincere way of showcasing your sexuality. We are not interested in cajoling or cheating. We are open within our community, but do not expect the same behavior in public or with non-swingers. So just because a beautiful woman is known to be a swinger does not mean that she will open her legs to anyone. We (women) are the ones in control most of the time. We are in control and command respect. The smart men know that women are the ones that make it happen (or kill it), so they are loyal and respectful.

Years later, when I no longer had a loving partner, I was often invited to swingers' parties, which I attended a couple of times. My experiences were different. Consequently, I learned a new aspect for my psyche, a prerequisite of my sexual being. Although I very much enjoyed fucking and eating pussy, I did not feel whole; I felt empty and thus did not get the satisfaction that I got in the past when my "loving" partner was present. This experience added reinforcement to my original belief in what a swinger's experience is—just recreational fun, an additional form of our own sexual high. On the surface, a swingers' event seems full of wonderful friends and loving relationships, but there is emotional disconnection. It is similar to when you watch a pornographic film. It is exciting and so much fun, but you are not emotionally connected to the actors. Thus, if we are not emotionally content, stable, and confident with ourselves and with our partners, then it will not be a great experience.

I realized I needed to be emotionally connected to a loving human being; man or woman (I thought). I enjoyed pussy and, for a while, I thought I was bisexual. As defined in Wikipedia, "bisexuality is romantic attraction, sexual attraction, or sexual behavior toward both males and females, or romantic or sexual attraction to people of any sex or gender identity."[39] I joined a bisexual group and tried to make connections, but I could not. I later learned that my psychological makeup did not allow me to court or answer to courting by a woman. This is another aspect of my sexual being . . . I am not bisexual . . . I am just kinky! And I feel no shame. I let shame go a long time ago.

Since then, I have not participated in any more sexual activities with the group. The opportunity did not present itself, and I did not go out of my way to find it. I realized that being bisexual is not a qualifier for swinging or being sexually promiscuous. I recognized that I was not looking for a relationship (with a woman). I just wanted to eat pussy.

Some friendships developed from my experience with the group, and we still stay in contact. Several of my friends classified themselves as polyamorous. When I met the term, I had to research to find a written explanation; my friends' explanations were great, but I needed an unbiased source. According to Wikipedia,[40] polyamory is the practice of, or desire for, intimate relationships where individuals may have more than one partner, with the knowledge and consent of all partners. It has been described as "consensual, ethical, and responsible non-monogamy." Although I thoroughly understand the concept, I do not relate to it at all. If I form a connection with my lover, he becomes my chosen partner, which stops me from bonding with another man; if I bond with a woman, then I cannot eat her pussy because that feels incestuous to me. My mind is geared to be a heterosexual female, but I also have a very sensual appreciation for the female body and a kinky need for pussy; and currently, it is all on hold.

I have been without a "loving" partner for a while, yet I feel no need to comply with invitations to swing, no need to please old acquaintances. They have tried to convince me with phrases like "enjoy life while you can," "life is too short," "you have to enjoy yourself," "enjoy yourself while you are young and pretty." The latter phrase was from someone much older (as I am no spring chicken), but to them, I am young. I agree with all those statements; I believe in enjoying life while I still can. However, my emotional state does not allow me to be in the mood for swinging. I yearn for a "loving" partner. I know that when I am happily involved in a loving relationship, I will be happy to swing again . . . if that is acceptable to my partner (. . . sigh!).

49.   Ebony Lust with a Fist

Okay, enough about the self-analysis. The exciting parts are my self-discovery. The first time I met with the group, I was ridiculously hot and eager for pussy. I met some beautiful and very feminine women. One tall, voluptuous black woman stood in the middle of the living room, raised her top, and said something along the lines of "I know ya'll want some of this. Come on, its ok." I was sure she read my mind or at least saw my desire in my face. I did want a taste and more. I walked up to her and started licking and sucking those nipples while gently squeezing her very firm and full breasts. Standing tall I was the perfect height—her tits were at mouth level. Still sucking, my hands traveled all around her ass and pussy. We soon moved to the couch and completely forgot about the room full of women watching us. As she sat on the couch, I spread her legs wide and raised her skirt inviting myself to her ebony treasure box. We were conveniently dressed as the theme was back to school. As I buried my face in her pussy and kept licking, savoring that clit, I felt someone raise my skirt and touch my ass. I made myself more inviting by bending on my knees in a wider stance and sticking my ass out for better reach. The gentle hand maneuvered with ease and efficacy making me even hotter. The feeling of her hand in my pussy kept getting fuller, more powerful and impactful. My whole bottom, pussy, ass, uterus, felt vibrating. I later realized that was me vibrating because of what she was doing. That was my first fisting experience, and it was awesome.

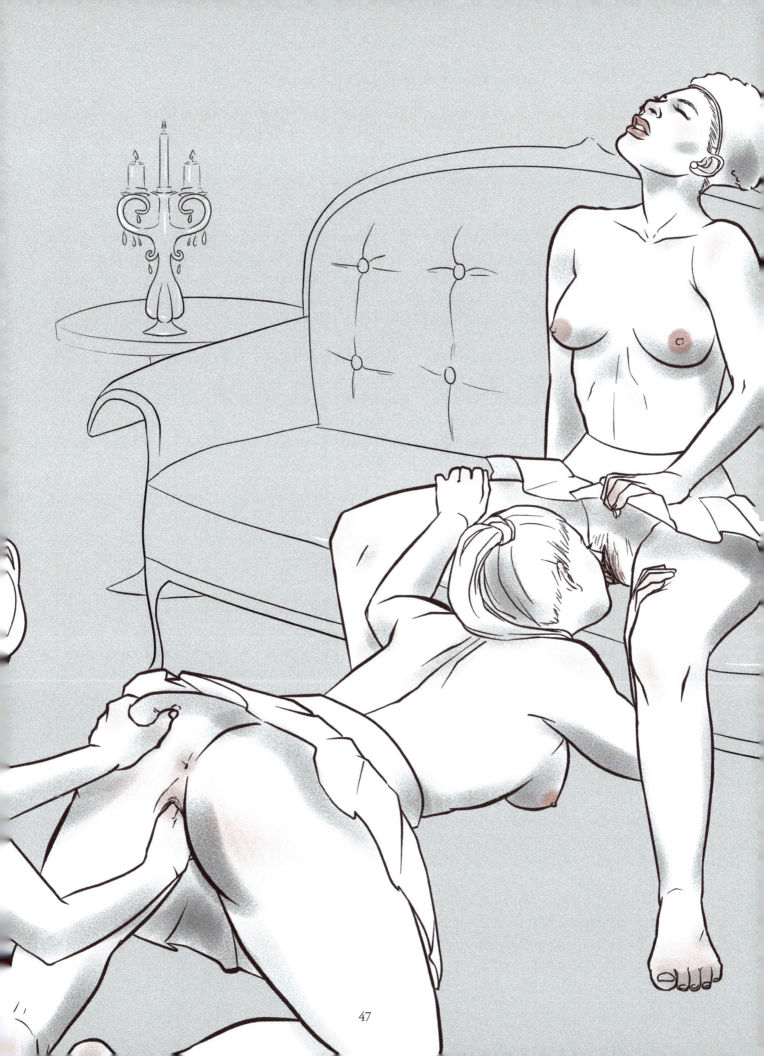

50. "He Who Controls Everything, Enjoys Nothing"

A few years ago, swinging with my boyfriend was going full force. I allowed him to be the "event planner," but I was always the one in charge. Most of the happy couples in the swinging community tend to do the same. It is also extremely important to discuss boundaries and to be careful not to overstep them. Most importantly, you and your partner must not arrive at the party with any issues of trust, resentment, or physical and emotional insecurity.

I would lie if I said I did not have to deal with those concerns at the beginning of our swinging excursions. It took some time, but I realized that it was due to my insecurity and mistrust of my partner. If you are not feeling secure in your relationship, if you do not feel fully accepted as the only one for your partner, then you will be in doubt that, when he fucks someone else, it is just recreational fun. You will fear that the minuscule emotional connection you share with him will culminate in the realization that he enjoys fucking someone else.

If you feel insecure about your beauty, then it will be difficult to let go and enjoy the presence of another naked female in the room. It is up to us to work through our issues, and my recommendation is honest communication within yourself and between you and your partner. If you still cannot work them out, then a professional is recommended. Unfortunately, many of us just let go of the relationship without taking a deep evaluation of our motives, desires, and fears. Often it is painful to grow and evolve, but if you see pain or discomfort as an inevitable and necessary part of the process then it will be easier to manage.

Note: This is not a book about relationships, and I am one of the many who could use some advice on the issue. I am simply stating my opinion.

51. The Pussy Buffet

The most memorable swingers' event I attended was full of bikers and leather princesses. I was dressed in a wet look (front) with straps on the back of the dress as well as cuffs with chains that tied to my leather choker. Yes, it was hot just to look at me but not because of my "natural beauty"—the outfit was enticing. I felt the feminine power, yet I can see how feminists would consider this a subservient uniform. It depends on how you take it. I have the power to say no, to do, and to take what I want. I utilized the chains to wrap around cocks as I teased them. The cold of the chains with the warm of my licks kept them in constant attention mode, reminiscent of little soldiers saluting the general. I made my way to a cute, petite, long-haired, Latin pussy, and we started enjoying one another's bodies while kissing. I asked her to get on top of the bar, which was very solid and just the right height for a delicious entrée of hot pussy. She happily complied, and I did not delay in savoring her cunt, but I did stop for a second to take a good look at her medium-rare style cunt. Yes, pink in the middle and a little darker around the edges of her inner lips with a swollen clit that looked like a sweet pink almond; delicious! That sight has stayed imprinted on my mind…three years later I still picture it and I savor it. I guess we were very loud with our humming because people started to gather around. During the heavy pussy licking and fingering, I noticed that another beautiful woman to my right was so into it, so I asked her to also sit on the bar. As soon as she did, I moved on to her, and that was the beginning of the pussy buffet. Men started picking up some women and sat them on the bar. Other women joined in the pussy eating, and the men started fucking us from behind. For a while, we were all eating and fucking in blissful unison.

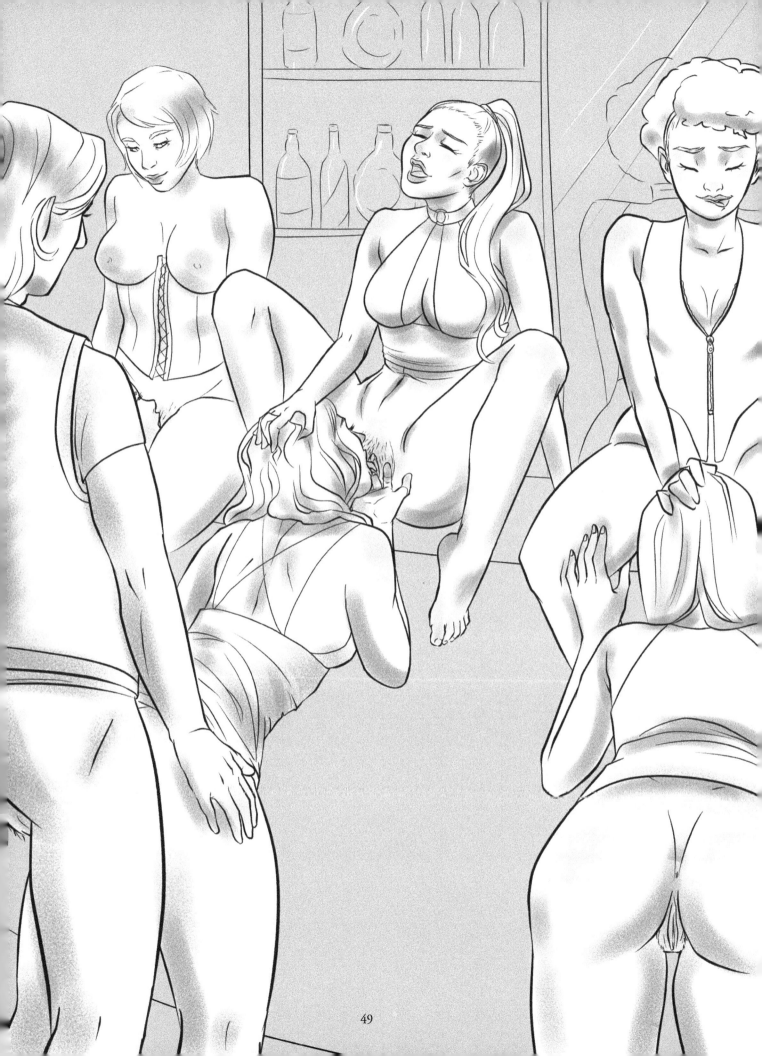

Most of my swinging occasions involved only one or two other couples. A small group is more comforting for the "newbies" and the shy, and it can be more pleasurable as there is less of a danger of getting left behind or neglected. It is also better to be with one couple who is gentle and comforting to the beginner's needs. I was lucky to have met wonderful people that were all that and more.

52. No Lover Left Behind

During the larger events (orgies), I often had to encourage my boyfriend to step into action. He was always very respectful and waited for invitations. In large groups, there will always be someone waiting to take a turn; if you are not careful, you may leave without getting any action.

I was not always this sympathetic; my partner taught me, mostly by example and extreme patience, not to be a selfish lover. On every occasion, he made sure I was pleased; he confirmed that I was ok with meeting new people. I started to do the same for him after a few experiences where he was accidentally left out. During these events as a woman, you will get so much attention that you may be distracted and assume that your partner is equally active. Keep attentive and do not leave him behind.

53. Find a Unicorn

If you are really into pussy eating, then the most gratifying option is inviting another bisexual woman to join you and your partner. For me, this is a favorite as it best suits my needs. And trust me when I say that a smart man will fully enjoy the view of two hot women with their legs open in V's rubbing their juice dripping pussies to exhilaration. At first try, this may be an awkward position but when you entangle your legs and your pussies meet, you will follow your instinct and rub like a pro.

54. Horseback Riding with a Twist

A slightly cool night with the brightest moonlight is perfect for some horseback riding. First, he mounts the horse (naked or with an open crotch); then you mount him. Begin with a slow rhythmic strut and increase as you please; not only is this romantic, it is truly exhilarating. A prerequisite is that he cannot be too big so that you can fully take him in or else you will be hurting at every step. Second, the horse must be strong enough for two people riding it.

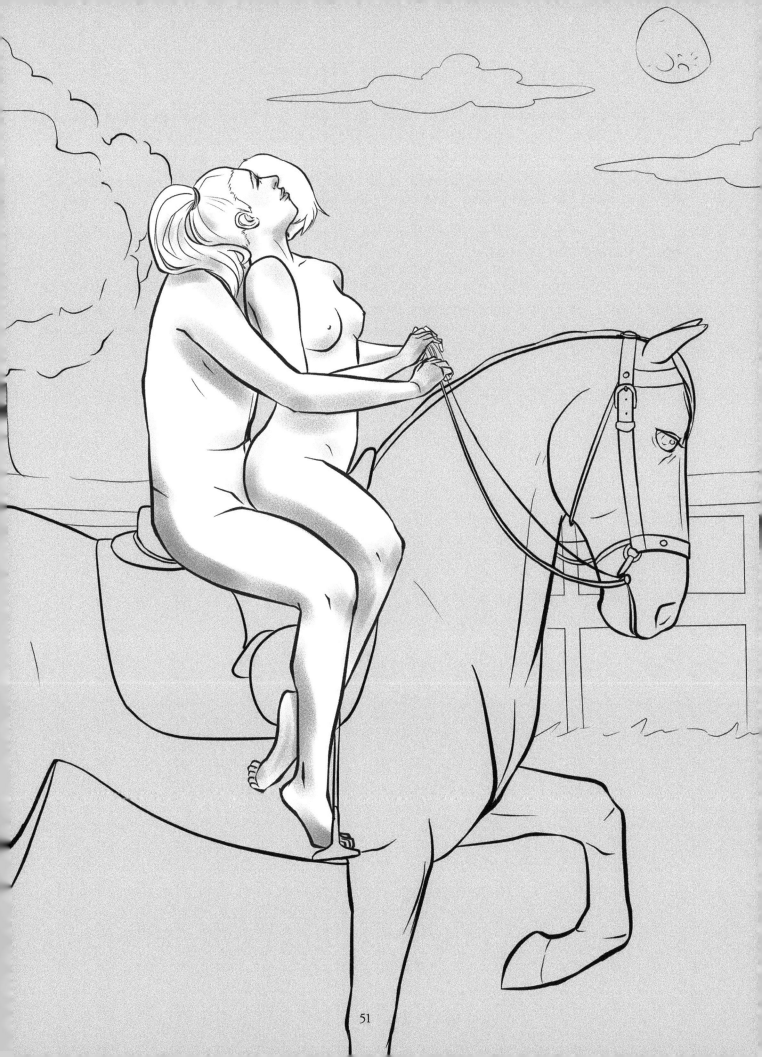

55. Allow for a Fetish

I do not know much about fetishes; I do not have any. I simply cannot relate or understand how a physical item could cause sexual excitement. However, I understand human beings enough to know that if your partner has a fetish, the loving response would be to allow it during the sexual encounters unless it is hurtful in any way. Loving yourself is communicating your fetish needs and to trying to incorporate it into your sexual lives. Again, situations like these require true communication and loving understanding by all in a relationship.

56. Pinned and Devoured

My favorite recollection of being pinned was by a male lover who grabbed me from behind; his arms holding back my arms. His legs wrapped around mine spreading them open to expose my fully aroused, juicy cunt. His girlfriend, who was very hungry for pussy, buried her face in mine and I was in ecstasy within seconds.

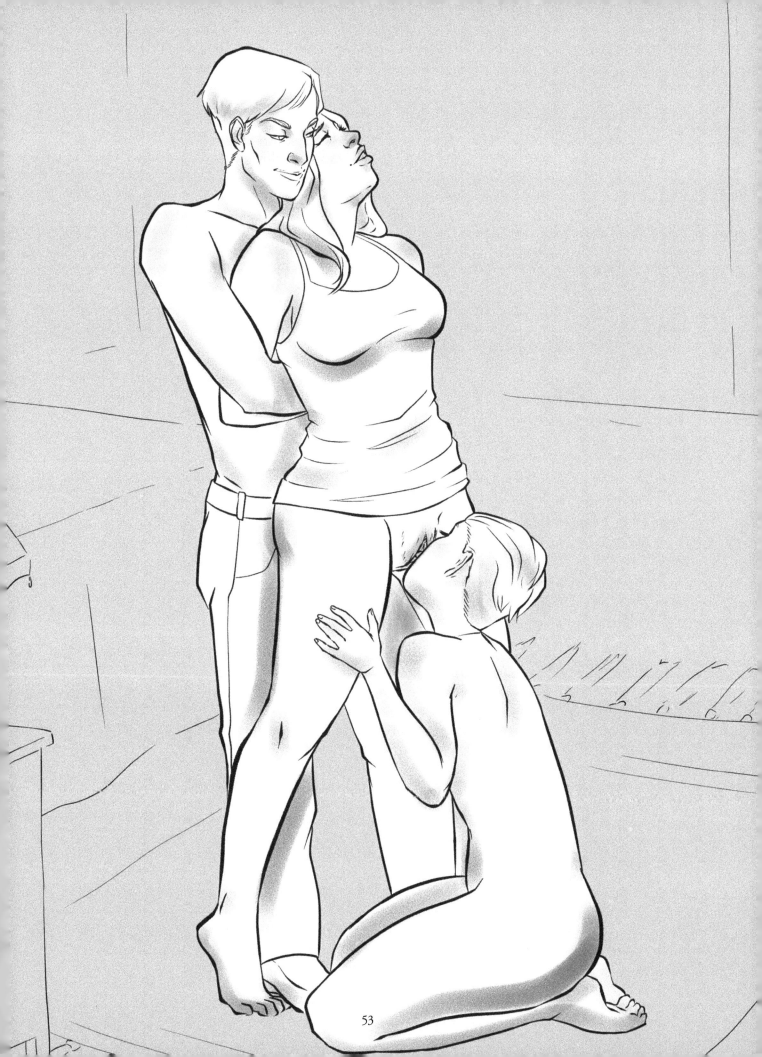

57. Silky Tongue Lashing

After I came several times, she then proceeded to insert a bullet vibrator in me and continued to lick me very gently, so gently that it was the most unimaginable silky feeling on my super engorged cunt. I kept coming, and coming, to the point where not only were my PC muscles contracting but also the lower part of my abdomen. It was unforgettable.

58. Banana Split Sunday

I had a surprise one Sunday morning when my boyfriend invited one of our friends/lovers over for brunch. We had a light crepe and fruit breakfast with some fun conversation. We quickly moved on to the luscious carpet where he had placed a bowl with fruits and whipped crème. She and I started playing with his luscious cock, enjoying the crème first by rubbing it from his cock back to his anus; then licking it off. We moved on to each other with the crème over our pussies and then licking it off while he watched. The Sunday sunlight coming through the window emitted an ethereal aura that added to our senses.

59. Double Fucking Renata

While he fucked her in her slightly elevated ass as she laid back on the ottoman, I lovingly kissed her and plunged a condom-covered banana into her pussy; this added a tightness that they both could feel making it more enjoyable. I did not need to add lubricant. Renata was so wet I could feel it while I fingered her before fucking her with the banana.

Another note, the banana was complete with its peel on and was ripe to a point of softness but strong enough to withstand her tight pussy.

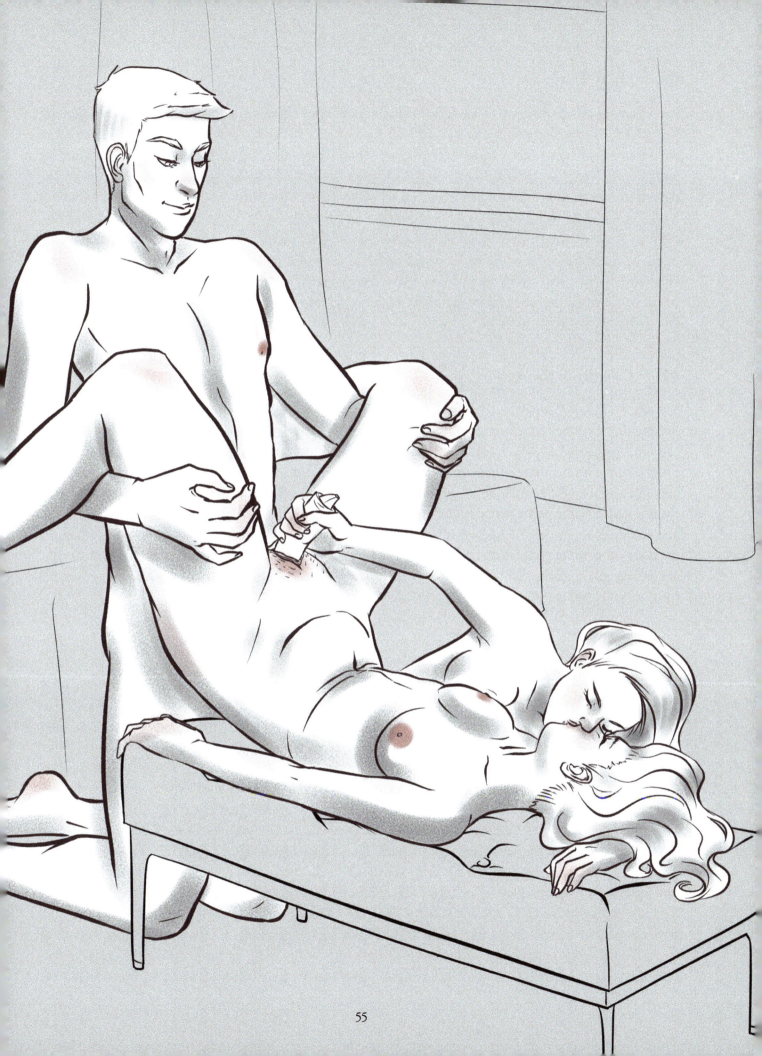

60.   Dirty Dancing

I met a couple for the first time at a local bar/club for drinks and conversation; it was safe, to a certain extent. I enjoyed their company and as time passed, I felt more at ease. When the music started, we got up to dance and I was quickly sandwiched between them. As her boobs met mine and his hard cock rubbed against my ass, I began to get hot. He had a long reach; he brought his hand under my skirt and up to my pussy. She danced so close to feel my boobs plump up and she spilled a bit of her drink on them, then proceeded to lick it off. She was quick as we did not want to bring too much attention to ourselves and risk getting kicked out. He kept gently rubbing my pussy and since my flowing skirt had plenty of material, it was not obvious. They were so natural and always smiling; I am sure they had done this before. Their easy-going, casual style was effective. My pussy was creaming, and I started to also grab her as well; casually rubbing her breasts, her ass. My arms were too short, but I wanted to also reach for her pussy, so I indicated I wanted to go back to our seat. I was hot and ready to fuck.

61.   Caught in the Act

Because we were still at the club, we had to mind our manners and be discrete. Again, I was sandwiched in our booth, which was a perfect spot for under-the-table foreplay. As we refreshed our lips with our drinks, she and I proceeded to kiss. She was succulent. Her lips reminded me of a hot cunt eager to be licked. She puckered up with her tongue in the middle, imitating a clit. I licked her imaging I was eating her pussy. He kept himself busy. As I turned to her, my ass was slightly turned sideways allowing him to lift my skirt all the way up (but still under the table) and take his cock out to feel me. Oh, he was hard. He wanted it bad and was ready to give it. Discretely this went on for a few minutes…we had to compose ourselves when the manager came to introduce himself and say hello. He knew what we were doing, and he said that usually, the special guests like ourselves move on to the upper level where we could enjoy special treats. We took the hint and paid the tab and walked upstairs to the VIP Room.

62.   Rumble in Booth #8

The entrance to the VIP Room was mysterious. A long but very narrow stairway led to an apple red door. I noticed the public entrance was on the opposite side. Next time we could just skip the vanilla bar and head straight to the swingers lifestyle club. The mood was a combination of sensual, nasty, and exciting. You could spot open cunts on the tables and their friend(s) taking turns. You could see a woman with a cock in her pussy, a cock in her ass, and a cock in her mouth. All very into themselves and each other. A hot, slender, long-haired woman was dancing on her table for her friend. While intently looking around, we found our way to booth #8; this was a more open half-oval shape. The back was low; you could not hide what you were doing, and that was ok. We did not want to hide. The exposure made it more exciting. We quickly got some ice and drinks (non-alcoholic by law) and got back to our fondling. Being in the middle, I pushed her back and started to lick her breasts and worked my way down to her pussy. As I did, I propped up my ass and he quickly lifted my skirt, pulled his cock right out, and started fucking me. He was very controlled. He fucked and fucked but did not come. After I made her come several times with my strong licking and finger probing of her g-spot, we sat up and got him in the middle for some cock sucking, taking turns on him. Again, he was still holding extraordinarily strong. We each took turns riding him, and throughout the taking turns, we all kissed and touched each other. I licked and sucked on her tits while she was riding him; she did the same as I rode him and squeezed him as if I wanted to choke his cock with my pussy. Then it was my turn. She pushed me down and started licking my pussy. He went behind her and started fucking her. She was an expert. I came so many times as she licked me and fucked me with her gentle yet firm fingers. She would not only go in and out but would circle, especially at the entrance of my pussy. We ate pussy and cock and fucked until dawn.

63. Chocolate Anus Lick for All

My favorite chocolates (Lindt Lindor Truffles, as I previously mentioned) have a hard exterior that when it breaks the liquid inside spills out. I love to rub it all over my lover's cock, balls, and anus; then lick and lick and lick and lick and lick and lick . . . it all off. I know he especially enjoys me licking his anus. That is a special need that I believed we should explore deeper (pun intended). Using chocolate helps those sensitive beings who can still smell the very distinct anus smell even if it is shiny clean. Our female guests were always enticed and loved the chocolate licking.

64. Exploring My Lover's Needs

As I planned, we explored, and my suspicions were correct; my lover did like the anus licking and mild finger penetration. I suggested and convinced him to go a step further. While buffing around his beautiful cock, I whispered in his ear, "Would you like to fuck and be fucked at the same time?" He got even harder; I thought his cock was going to explode. I continued: "Baby, just imagine, I lay down with my cunt propped up a little, you are penetrating my juicy hot pussy, and then . . . you feel these robust hands grab a stronghold of your ass and open to expose your sweet little anus . . . then slowly he licks to prime you for more. Then you feel the cock coming in, forcing itself into you, pushing through…then he grabs a hold of your hips as he thrusts and your cock gets a stronghold in my wet pussy, and he thrusts again, and again my pussy contracts, he thrusts, and thrusts, and thrusts. . ." My partner had a grand finish, spraying his cum all over my face.

65. A Step Further

The next step was to see if he would enjoy the actual penetration. At first, we tried fucking him with dildos and butt plugs. He enjoyed the hot sex talk, replaying the scene of fucking while being fucked. I could see his excitement so I knew that we could go a step further.

66. To Fuck and Be Fucked (in unison)

Soon after, he worked up the courage to agree to actual penetration from a real cock. He searched and searched until the day came that he met someone that agreed to meet us. He was a young banker who was in incredibly good physical shape; he was only interested in male fucking, and that was ok with me. My focus was on my lover. We met at a hotel and had a few drinks to break the ice. When he went to the bathroom, my lover took advantage of his absence to get me started. He undressed me, kissed me, took me to the bed, and started fucking me. When our guest came out, he was ready; only wearing a G-string with an opening for his cock. I barely got a glimpse because he wasted no time. I could feel it when he started touching my lover from behind because my lover's cock was bigger than I had ever felt. His humming became a little louder and his facial expression a little more dramatic. Then the trusting began, slow, slow, slow, then it picked up speed but not too much. Our guest was savoring the task and took his time. My lover was relishing fucking and being fucked at the same time. I could sense that as he gripped on to me and his cock stayed so firm and hot throughout until we reached climax. I had come several times already, but our guest was polite to finish in unison with my lover. We all finished with a great smiles and very loud sighs. It was good for me, and I know that it was incredible for my lover. We finished our drinks and said goodbye. I knew that we would do this again, and that was ok with me. If you wonder how am I loving myself on such occasions, I assure you that I inherently like to explore and I want to be happy with my lover; therefore, exploring my lover's sexuality is part of exploring for my pleasure.

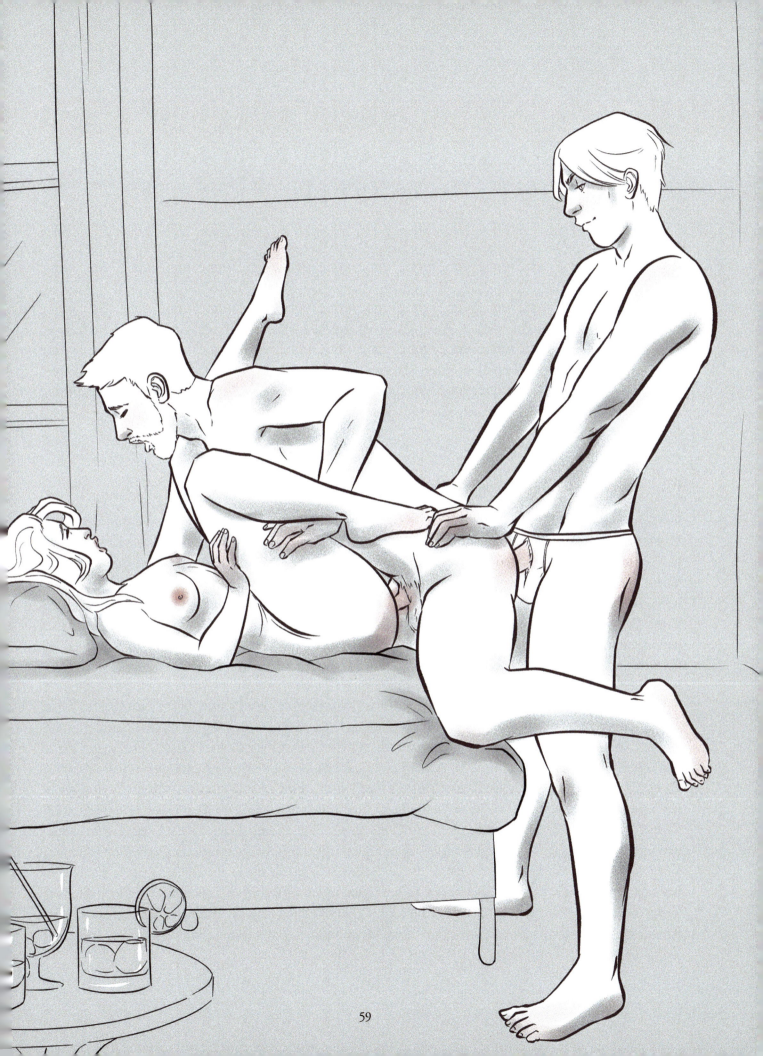

SECTION V
Set the Standards

The male (body as well as the soul) is also under many societal constraints. Those constraints also affect our relationships with men, for we cannot be fully free until they are free. If it is ok for them to accept their sensuality, vulnerability, and emotional need, then we will have better relationships because then we can meet at the same level. They are, I believe, even more vulnerable than us women. As I mentioned at the beginning of this book, we can endure extremely high emotional and physical pain. I believe that we can help them be free by example.

67. Foster an Equal Mentality

Needless to mention, I am a feminist. I think I was born that way, which is surprising as I was raised in a Hispanic/Catholic culture from childhood to my early teens. In first grade, my teacher asked me to write one page of my mother's name and one page of my father's name. In the Latin/Hispanic culture, the women's name is usually the first name, maiden name 'of' Husband's last name, culturally indicating she belongs to her husband. Well, I did exactly that. When I wrote my father's name, I did the same: First name, Last name, "of" mother's last name. I was corrected by the teacher. The correct way was just his first name and his paternal and maternal last names, but to me, that sounded like unfair treatment. If my mother "belonged" to my father, then my father "belonged" to my mother—that was the fair treatment in my little 6-year-old brain.

We need to foster our "equal" mentality. Many times I witnessed my mother sacrificing her time, her food, and her health for my father and her children. I admit I did not want to fall prey to that culture of self-sacrifice, but I realize how important it is to have the nurturing that she gave us. However, the weight of the responsibility of nurturing needs to be done by both parents, or our view of parenting roles will always be skewed. But how do we begin this trend? This is a long journey which we can start with small but impactful things. One example is how we often compliment little girls with adjectives like pretty, beautiful, clean, obedient, and responsible. We often compliment boys on how fast, strong, smart, or tough they are. In reality, they can both be tough, smart, and beautiful, so let's not gender limit the compliments. In the article "Sexism and Parenting: Protect Your Girls & Boys," Julian Redwood explains the two main areas where we need to work on. The first is to look at ourselves and be honest about our own sexist beliefs so that we can reduce the impact on our children. Second, deal with the sexism around us and help the children analyze the situation. Redwood points out that as parents, we come across situations where we must use the opportunity to explain the underpinnings of the images or reactions that our children see.[41]

I am so grateful and lucky that my father tried to educate us to be self-sufficient to avoid dependence on men. He knew well how his society accepted the subjugation of women, and he did not want that kind of life for his daughters. He also took opportunities to explain some of the societal images and comments to expose the irrationality in sexism. I recall a beer commercial in which a woman finishes her work shift and puts away her welding gear, then she enjoys a beer. My brother said, "These women are somewhat 'tasteless,'" referring to the working woman on the screen. My father replied, "You think that because these women no longer have to put up with a man's beating or insults. They don't need him because they can now support themselves." Yes, my brother was very "traditional" and on occasions, our belief systems clashed. My father also took time to explain the difference between being religious and being spiritual; that we did not have to blindly obey a priest or person of authority; that respect is earned, not obediently given; and, most importantly, that the best place to worship God is in your heart, not the church. By fostering an equal mentality, we become aware when someone is intending to treat us, women, as second-class citizens.

Unfortunately, when a young girl reaches puberty, many parents approach this time terrified. As a result, most of the conversations are about "not getting pregnant"; there are many variations of this topic, but the only message that reaches her is "no SEX, no SEX, no SEX." What we should be doing is talking about contraception and bringing to light all the possibilities for her future; the possibilities for her career or vocational training, and her options to live at home or start preparing to be on her own. By creating a brighter outlook of her future, she will be more careful about engaging in sexual encounters.

During my teenage years, all I heard was to not have sex; there was never discussion or support for a better future. All that talk made me think that my best chance of having a good future was to find a husband who would provide it. These years were challenging because the pressure was coming from my father. It was confusing and ironic because, in the past, he was outspoken about making sure that we educate ourselves, that we learn some skill to be self-sufficient so that we would not fall prey to a marriage forged by necessity. So when I reached that late "teenagehood," it felt as if his logic deserted him and he succumbed to the traditional beliefs that a woman loses value once she's been sexually active. I rebelled, for my spirit could not yield to such deprecating circumstances. I kept working and going to school and was careful not to get pregnant because that would make life even more difficult for me. How could I support a child when I could barely support myself? I wanted a career, a profession, so I was well aware that a child would make my goals much more difficult to reach.

68. Demand Respect

Respect is something that we must learn and demand, even if we think our demands will go unheard. To some it is common to hear catcalls and shrug them off, thinking "boys will be boys." This is an example of accepting a situation that is humiliating to a woman. At the age of 13, I had just recently arrived in the U.S. That summer, I spent the afternoons riding my bike. I enjoyed getting to know the neighborhood; I enjoyed the freedom, the newness of it all. We lived in an 8-unit apartment complex—2 rows of 4 units each with parking on the ground level and living quarters upstairs. I have always been a quiet, reserved person, even more so in my childhood. Across from our apartment, to the opposite corner, there lived several young men who were also Hispanic. They knew my brothers, but I had never spoken to them. One hot afternoon as I finished my rounds on my bike, much to my surprise, I heard a man call my name followed by some loud kisses. I turned, threw my bike down with force, and yelled at the group of men sitting on the stairs of that apartment *"Hijo de tu chingada Madre, ven aqui a decirme eso y te arranco los huevos con mis uñas,"* which translates to "Son of a bitch, come here and tell me that and I will rip your balls off with my fingernails!"

My demeanor changed to match the strength of my character. I was no longer the shy little woman they saw. I was strong, and my stance was like a tiger ready to pounce and rip the balls off my target. The young man who threw the kisses was surprised and ran upstairs while his friends made fun of him. They never bothered me after that. I am sure that if I had not spoken up, if I had taken the insult, they would have continued.

Later in my late twenties, while working in the male-dominated alcoholic beverage industry, I had to once again demand respectful treatment. I worked with inept and unqualified managers. There was nothing I could do about that; however, when I was horrendously disrespected due to my hearing disability, I went for the jugular. I wrote a long letter to the owner in which I explained how a co-worker had made fun of my hearing disability in front of my immediate supervisor who just sat there complicit. I explained to him how uneducated, unqualified middle management is putting his company in danger of very damaging lawsuits. I had no desire to sue, as I enjoyed my work, but I was not about to let that atrocity go unnoticed. That action did not win me any friends, but at least they were careful about how they treated me going forward.

So how am I loving myself? Standing up for myself. Refusing to accept disrespectful treatment is loving yourself. No matter the size of the crowd, no matter how nervous you may feel, it is important that we value ourselves more than the opinions of others. Those who bully will not take on the ones that will be strong and fight to "death" in battle. Facing your aggressor from the beginning is essential to establish yourself as a fearless warrior, and they will think twice before starting a battle with a fearless Goddess.

Note: Please consider that there are those women who will be helpless no matter what they do and that is unfortunate. It makes a huge difference when we have the support of family and community so that we feel strong enough to stand our ground. I have never experienced being a victim of sexual harassment or abuse. It could be that from the beginning, I came across as a strong woman (in mind and body), or it could be that I have been lucky. I strongly believe that a predator looks for those who fear him or trust him. I have not done either and have always remained in control of myself—meaning no drugs, limited alcohol, and never leaving my drinks unattended. If I let loose, it is because I *want* to fuck; but for a predator, there is no fun in that.

69. Education is the Best Equalizer

As mentioned earlier, more women than men are obtaining higher-level degrees, and that will help women assume more powerful positions in government and industry. But my reference to education is not just the typical college education. It is important for women, especially those who do not excel academically, to know basic things like how to create their budget, to do a simple tax return, to change a tire, to mow the lawn, to know simple plumbing, and yes, even how to prepare a simple meal. Vocational training can be a lifesaver for the disadvantaged because that can be the floater to get you to the next level. Wherever you work, learn everything you can about your job. Assist others and learn about their job. This practice will help you reach other opportunities and will make your life much richer in general.

You also owe it to yourself to know your sexual being—our sexual drive is the strongest drive following our survival instinct. It is this drive that hides behind the mask of love and can wreak havoc in our lives. Our unchecked drive for sexual satisfaction can lead us to unattended children (for which they suffer consequences), destroy loving relationships, and it can even drive us to murder. How can this be? The simplest of examples is the case of Amy Fisher and her assassination attempt on her lover's wife, Mary Jo Buttafuoco. I was still an impressionable young woman when this case came on the news. This was the first time I realized how sex can drive us to commit actions that can wreck our lives. Again, I remind you that I am no scientist; my writing is simply my opinion, so here it goes. In the case of young Amy, 16, having sex with a 34-year-old man was a crime in itself; behind the age gap, there is the **Sexual Experience gap**—that is the real danger. Sexual experience can be a powerful weapon, a controlling force over the inexperienced. This is another reason why masturbation, making love to yourself, is so important. If the woman can only experience sexual pleasure when a man is touching her, then she depends on men for something so beautiful, so essential, and this can be extremely dangerous. We need to teach our daughters to love themselves physically and emotionally.

The most important education, however, is to learn about yourself; learn what inspires you and what heals you. In the process, you will learn and create "the highest, truest, expression of yourself" Oprah Winfrey.

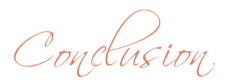

Conclusion

Our sexuality is our vehicle to sensual and spiritual connection to our lover(s). We all know the dangers of driving a car. The statistics that you will be in an auto-related accident are overwhelming. Does that well-known fact stop us from driving or riding in a vehicle? No. We would be miserable. So, we take precautions. We take driving lessons. We use our seat belts. We drive at considerate speeds. We drive courteously. We follow the driving guidelines established by the law. We try to ride only with careful drivers.

Many of us do the same when dealing with sexual relations. We use condoms (for men and women), and we try to select partners who are as selective as we are. We make sure that there is no opening in our skin (such as cuts, pimples, etc.), which would allow bacteria or viruses easy access to our internal bodies. We also get medical checkups so that we do not pass on infections if we do have any.

The one especially important thing we are missing is the "driving lessons." It is almost unheard of to give teenagers or young adults lessons about our sexuality and, much less, our sensuality. I believe that is wrong. We are not bringing to light one of the major characteristics of our humanity. If there had been a class, a teacher to learn from, I would have reached the wisdom of sexual/sensual relations much sooner than my forty-fifth birthday; so many years squandered trying to find my way without a compass, without my sexuality "owner's manual."

For centuries, women have been held as property. Their lack of sexual experience and "purity" or "impurity" was the determinant of their value (or lack of). This way of living keeps women "under control" until our vast dam of sexual desire breaks loose. If we are not taught how to control our sexual drive, we are bound to make horrendous mistakes or lose our minds to anxiety, depression, and other psychological traumas. This also applies to men, of course, but they have not been bound to ridiculous standards of sexual restraint as women have been, nor have they been so humiliated and punished by society for breaking any sexual behavior standards.

The teachings of self-love, masturbation, and sexual enlightenment will strengthen the student and will help in their wise selection of a loving partner, spouse, mate, or whatever it is that they are looking for. Although sex is a powerful force, we all still yearn to be loved, and that is another powerful force within us. Gaining control over our sexual drive will enable us to be patient and selective in finding a genuinely loving partner.

Even though my self-acceptance didn't come shining to the surface till my middle-age years—and I admit it sounds a bit sad—I am so happy to be aware of my sexual self as I am now in my older years. I look forward to old age because I know that my sexuality will still be there and, with a resourceful and creative mind like mine, I am also confident that I will live a fabulous sensual and sexual life.

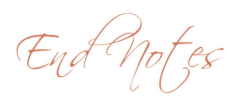

1. https://en.wikipedia.org/wiki/Levator_ani#Pubococcygeus
2. https://en.wikipedia.org/wiki/Dopamine
3. https://en.wikipedia.org/wiki/Operant_conditioning
4. *Chiras DD (2012). Human Biology (7th ed.). Sudbury, MA: Jones & Bartlett Learning. p. 262. ISBN 978-0-7637-8345-7*
5. *Blaicher W, Gruber D, Bieglmayer C, Blaicher AM, Knogler W, Huber JC (1999). "The role of oxytocin in relation to female sexual arousal". Gynecologic and Obstetric Investigation. 47 (2): 125–6. PMID 9949283. doi:10.1159/000010075.*
6. *Anderson-Hunt M, Dennerstein L (1995). "Oxytocin and female sexuality". Gynecologic and Obstetric Investigation. 40 (4): 217–21. PMID 8586300. doi:10.1159/000292340.*
7. *Murphy MR, Seckl JR, Burton S, Checkley SA, Lightman SL (October 1987). "Changes in oxytocin and vasopressin secretion during sexual activity in men". The Journal of Clinical Endocrinology and Metabolism. 65 (4): 738–41. PMID 3654918. doi:10.1210/jcem-65-4-738.*
8. *Krüger TH, Haake P, Chereath D, Knapp W, Janssen OE, Exton MS, Schedlowski M, Hartmann U (April 2003). "Specificity of the neuroendocrine response to orgasm during sexual arousal in men". The Journal of Endocrinology. 177 (1): 57–64. PMID 12697037. doi:10.1677/joe.0.1770057.*
9. *Goldstein I, Meston CM, Davis S, Traish A (17 November 2005).* Women's Sexual Function and Dysfunction: Study, Diagnosis and Treatment. *CRC Press. pp. 205–. ISBN 978-1-84214-263-9.*
10. Wiley Interdiscip Rev Cogn Sci. 2015 Sep-Oct;6(5):409-17. doi: 10.1002/wcs.1354. Epub 2015 Jun 22. https://www.ncbi.nlm.nih.gov/pubmed/26267407.
11. http://www.who.int/mediacentre/news/releases/2014/world-health-statistics-2014/en/
12. *https://www.ncbi.nlm.nih.gov/pmc/articles/PMC1432200/*
13. https://www.youtube.com/watch?time_continue=6&v=u4kvpjQe8nw
14. http://quodid.com/quotes/585/timothy-leary/women-who-seek-to-be-equal-with-men
15. Male babies http://www.sciencemag.org/news/2014/12/why-women-s-bodies-abort-males-during-tough-times
16. https://www.psychologytoday.com/blog/beautiful-minds/201207/men-women-and-iq-setting-the-record-straight.
17. https://en.wikipedia.org/wiki/Marilyn_vos_Savant
18. https://www.smithsonianmag.com/history/the-demonization-of-empress-wu-20743091/
19. https://www.historyextra.com/period/elizabethan/elizabeth-i-love-life-was-she-virgin-queen-robert-dudley-earl-essex/#:~:text=While%20foreign%20negotiations%20continued%2C%20Elizabeth,first%2C%20and%20probably%20only%20love.
20. https://www.biography.com/royalty/queen-elizabeth-i
21. https://www.britannica.com/biography/Cleopatra-queen-of-Egypt
22. http://www.ascentofwoman.com/1-civilisation
23. https://www.ancient.eu/Enheduanna/
24. https://www.britannica.com/biography/Theodora-Byzantine-empress-died-548
25. https://en.wikipedia.org/wiki/Mochizuki_Chiyome
26. https://en.wikipedia.org/wiki/Juana_Azurduy_de_Padilla
27. http://www.harriet-tubman.org/category/biography/
28. https://awpc.cattcenter.iastate.edu/directory/ernestine-l-rose/
29. https://www.biography.com/activist/ida-b-wells
30. https://en.wikipedia.org/wiki/Truus_Menger-Oversteegen
31. https://www.britannica.com/biography/Malala-Yousafzai
32. https://www.vanguardngr.com/2020/06/eight-years-after-shooting-nobel-prize-winner-malala-graduates/

33 https://video.search.yahoo.com/search/video?fr=mcafee&p=tarana+burke#id=1&vid=d6ba468c05226dff735d9de94c429577&action=click
34 https://en.wikipedia.org/wiki/Greta_Thunberg
35 https://news.yahoo.com/climate-activist-greta-thunberg-sail-101219927.html
36 https://www.msn.com/en-us/news/us/i-am-someone-s-daughter-too-read-rep-ocasio-cortez-s-full-speech-responding-to-rep-ted-yoho/ar-BB1795Hf
37 https://www.psychologytoday.com/us/blog/life-refracted/201902/learning-love-and-be-loved
38 https://www.psychologytoday.com/us/blog/married-and-still-doing-it/201708/what-sex-really-means-women
39 https://en.wikipedia.org/wiki/Bisexuality
40 https://en.wikipedia.org/wiki/Polyamory
41 https://goodmenproject.com/featured-content/sexism-parenting-protect-your-girls-boys-wcz/
42 https://en.wikipedia.org/wiki/Ruth_Bader_Ginsburg

CPSIA information can be obtained
at www.ICGtesting.com
Printed in the USA
BVHW022339170122
626473BV00004B/4

9 781665 548113